EMQs for Dentistry
Third edition

Douglas Hammond
BDS (Wales) MFGDP (UK) MFDS (London)
MOralSurg (London) MBBS (UCL)
MRCS (London) FRCS (London) PhD (UCLAN)

Barry Quinn
BDS, MSc, LDSRCS (Eng), MRDRCS (Ed),
FDSRCPS (Glas), FFDRCS (Irel), FHEA

Richard Moore
BDS, MFDS RCPS (Glasg),
MAcadMed, FRSPH, AIFL

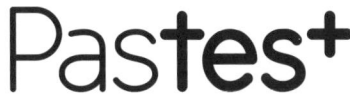

© 2016 Pastest Ltd
Egerton Court
Parkgate Estate
Knutsford
Cheshire
WA16 8DX

Telephone: 01565 752000

All rights reserved. No part of this publication may be reproduced, stored in a retrieval system, or transmitted, in any form or by any means, electronic, mechanical, photocopying, recording or otherwise without the prior permission of the copyright owner.

First Published 2007
Second Edition Published 2011
Third Edition Published 2016

ISBN: 978-1-905635-98-6
eISBN: 978-1-909491-92-2 MobiPocket
          978-1-909491-93-9 ePUB

A catalogue record for this book is available from the British Library.

The information contained within this book was obtained by the author from reliable sources. However, while every effort has been made to ensure its accuracy, no responsibility for loss, damage or injury occasioned to any person acting or refraining from action as a result of information contained herein can be accepted by the publishers or author.

Pastest Online Revision, Books and Courses

Pastest provides online revision, books and courses to help medical students and doctors maximise their personal performance in critical exams and tests. Our in-depth understanding is based on over 40 years' experience and the feedback of recent exam candidates.

Resources are available for:
Medical school applicants and undergraduates, MRCP, MRCS, MRCPCH, DCH, GPST, MRCGP, FRCA, Dentistry, and USMLE Step 1.

For further details contact:
Tel: 01565 752000   Fax: 01565 650264
www.pastest.com   enquiries@pastest.com

Text prepared in the UK by Carnegie Book Production, Lancaster
Printed and bound in the UK by Bell & Bain Ltd, Glasgow

Contents

About the Author		iv
Contributors to the third edition		v
Introduction		vi
Preface to the third edition		vi
1	Child Dental Health and Orthodontics	1
2	General Medicine	41
3	Oral Medicine	93
4	Oral Pathology	135
5	Oral Surgery	179
6	Periodontics	225
7	Pharmacology	257
8	Radiology	299
9	Restorative Dentistry and Materials	341
Index		381

About the Author

Douglas Hammond BDS (Wales) MFGDP (UK) MBBS (UCL) MRCS (London)

Douglas is a Senior Lecturer in Surgical Science and Consultant Oral and Maxillofacial Surgeon. Douglas graduated from Cardiff Dental Hospital and completed various hospital and practice jobs. He then spent four years working as a part-time lecturer in Oral and Maxillofacial Surgery whilst completing his medicine degree at University College London. His junior medical jobs were completed at Southampton, and specialist training in the West Midlands.

Contributors to the third edition

Barry Quinn BDS, MSc, LDSRCS (Eng), MRDRCS (Ed), FDSRCPS (Glas), FFDRCS (Irel), FHEA
Senior Specialist Clinical Teacher / Honorary Consultant at King's College London Dental Institute
Barry Quinn is an undergraduate lead for over 180 students at King's College London which includes a multi-professional teaching team of Specialist and General Dentists, Dental Therapists and Hygienists, Dental Nurses and Radiographers. Barry is an Honorary Consultant in Restorative Dentistry and Specialist in Prosthodontics. He is a curriculum lead for years 4/5 of the BDS programme and is academic lead for the Management and Leadership course. Barry is an examiner for the Royal College of Surgeons of England and Edinburgh as well as being an external examiner for the Dental Schools in Queen Mary's University of London, Belfast, Cardiff and Khartoum. He has been an OSCE lead for the Overseas Registration Examination as well as being an examiner and question writer for MJDF, MFDS and MRD.He has been awarded an ADEE mature educators award as well as the inaugural Inter-professional Educators award in 2016. His research has involved working with inter-professional teams in developing haptic simulation for dental, medical, nursing and veterinary professionals. He is a member of both ADEE and ADEA and is President elect for the Education Research Group of the IADR and President of the British Dental Association Metropolitan Branch (London). He has published over 100 articles including two books, exploring issues on inter-professionalism, simulation, technology enhance learning, sleep apnoea and the role of the Dental Team in identifying victims of domestic violence.
Barry has recently been invited by UNESCO to join the IFIP working group 3.3, Research into Educational Applications of Information Technologies.

Richard Moore BDS, MFDS RCPS (Glasg), MAcadMed, FRSPH, AIFL
Richard has worked exclusively in oral and maxillofacial surgery since graduating from the University of Birmingham in 2002. He has delivered and designed teaching programmes for postgraduate dentists in junior hospital posts in oral and maxillofacial surgery across the UK. He has also been involved in Residency programmes in Canada. Previous academic appointments include Kings College London and The University of Warwick Medical School; he also examines for the Royal College of Surgeons. Richard is currently the Programme Director for the Diploma in Oral Surgery at the Royal College of Surgeons England and holds a substantive post in Oral Surgery at Doncaster and Bassetlaw NHS Foundation Trust.

Introduction

EMQs are an interesting way of testing knowledge. They require a thorough grounding in each subject, and the large number of stems ensures that the ability to 'guess' the correct answer is reduced. However, EMQs are difficult to write in a way which enables the student to narrow down some subjects and the way in which they can be examined.

This book aims to cover a large number of topics which are commonly questioned in dentistry examinations. The answers and explanations should help students increase their knowledge and also identify areas which require more work. Hopefully this book will be a useful tool for revision.

Douglas Hammond

Preface to the third edition

This third edition has been thoroughly revised bringing the questions up to date and relevant for the current postgraduate dental examinations such as MJDF. The explanations have been revised to allow the book to be used as a revision aid as well as practice questions and is not only aimed at postgraduates and core trainees but also final year dental students.

Richard Moore

1
Child Dental Health and Orthodontics

1.1 Theme: Child Development

1.2 Theme: Childhood Illnesses

1.3 Theme: Chromosomal Abnormalities

1.4 Theme: International Caries Detection and Assessment System (ICDAS-II codes)

1.5 Theme: Trauma to the Primary Dentition

1.6 Theme: Tooth-brushing Techniques (1)

1.7 Theme: Dates of Eruption (1)

1.8 Theme: Dates of Eruption (2)

1.9 Theme: Dates of Eruption (3)

1.10 Theme: Dental Trauma (1)

1.11 Theme: Dental Trauma (2)

1.12 Theme: Behaviour Management

1.13 Theme: Tooth Size

1.14 Theme: Cephalometrics (1)

1.15 Theme: Cephalometrics (2)

1.16 Theme: Occlusion (1)

1.17 Theme: Occlusion (2)

1.18 Theme: Terminology

1.19 Theme: Dental Anomalies

1.20 Theme: Index of Orthodontic Treatment Needs (IOTN)

1.21 Theme: Fluoride

1.22 Theme: Tooth-brushing Techniques (2)

1.23 Theme: Cephalometrics (3)

1.24 Theme: Skeletal Relationships, Mandibular Positions and Paths of Closure

1.25 Theme: Treatment of Deciduous Teeth

1.26 Theme: Dates of Calcification

1.27 Theme: Malocclusion

1.28 Theme: General Paediatric Conditions

1.29 Theme: Dates of Eruption and Chronological Age

1.30 Theme: Abnormalities of Eruption

1.31 Theme: Abnormalities of Tooth Structure/Number

2 CHILD DENTAL HEALTH AND ORTHODONTICS

1.1 Theme: Child Development

A	2 months
B	4 months
C	6 months
D	9 months
E	12 months
F	18 months
G	24 months
H	36 months
I	48 months

From the list above, choose the age at which a normally developing child will be able to do each of the following activities. You may use each option once, more than once or not at all.

1. Build a tower of three cubes
2. Draw a circle
3. Hold a rattle and shake
4. Sit unsupported
5. Says 'mama'

1.2 Theme: Childhood Illnesses

A	Diphtheria
B	*Haemophilus meningitis*
C	Mumps
D	Pertussis
E	Polio
F	Rubella
G	Tuberculosis
H	Varicella zoster

From the above options, choose the most appropriate diagnosis for the clinical observations below. You may use each option once, more than once or not at all.

1. Anterior horn cell damage leading to paralysis may occur.
2. Developing fetus may develop cataracts, deafness and congenital heart disease, if the mother becomes infected.
3. Persistent productive cough, night sweats and weight loss.
4. Dry cough with characteristic 'whooping' noise.
5. Parotid gland enlargement, deafness and orchitis may occur.

1.3 Theme: Chromosomal Abnormalities

A 45 XO
B Trisomy 13
C Trisomy 18
D Trisomy 21
E Pierre-Robin sequence

From the above options, match each of the syndromes listed below with the chromosomal analysis. You may use each option once, more than once or not at all.

1 Down

2 Edward

3 Patau

4 Turner

1.4 Theme: International Caries Detection and Assessment System (ICDAS-II codes)

A 0
B 1
C 2
D 3
E 4
F 5
G 6

For each of the descriptions below, choose the correct ICDAS-II code option from the list above. You may use each option once, more than once or not at all.

1 Distinctive cavity with visible dentine.

2 Distinct visual change in enamel seen when wet.

3 Extensive distinct cavity (more than half the surface) with visible dentine.

4 First visual change in enamel: opacity or discoloration visible at a pit of fissure after prolonged drying.

5 Non-cavitated with underlying dark shadow from dentine.

1.5 Theme: Trauma to the Primary Dentition

- **A** Avulsion
- **B** Concussion
- **C** Crown fracture
- **D** Crown-root fracture
- **E** Extrusive luxation
- **F** Intrusive luxation
- **G** Lateral luxation
- **H** Root fracture
- **I** Subluxation

For each of the following clinical scenarios, choose the most appropriate option from the list above. You may use each option once, more than once or not at all.

1. A 4-year-old has fallen over and hit the upper right central incisor. On clinical examination the tooth is supra-occluded, and on radiographic examination a horizontal dark line is evident across the apical third of the root.

2. A toddler has tripped, and now the two central incisors are infra-occluded.

3. A 3-year-old boy has hit his mouth against a toy, and his mother has noticed that a tooth is chipped.

4. A 6-year-old girl has been knocked in the mouth playing. She now says that the upper left central incisor tooth is tender; on clinical examination the tooth is firm, and no radiographic changes are evident.

5. A 4-year-old girl has been hit in the face playing ball. The upper left lateral incisor is now supra-occluded. On clinical examination the tooth is mobile, and radiographically there is a widened periodontal ligament space.

1.6 Theme: Tooth-brushing Techniques (1)

A Apply pressure to blanch the gingivae, then remove. Repeat several times. Slightly rotate the brush and gradually move it occlusally
B Roll brush occlusally, maintaining contact with gingivae, then the tooth surface
C Scrub in antero-posterior direction, keeping brush horizontal
D Vibrate the brush, not changing the position of the bristles
E Vibrate the brush while moving it apically into the gingival margin
F With the teeth in occlusion, move the brush in a rotary motion against the maxillary and mandibular tooth surfaces and gingival margins

For each of the following tooth-brushing techniques, choose the option that describes the technique from the list above. You may use each option once, more than once or not at all.

1 Charter's
2 Bass
3 Stillman

1.7 Theme: Dates of Eruption (1)

A 0–3 months
B 3–6 months
C 6–9 months
D 9–12 months
E 12–15 months
F 15–18 months
G 18–21 months
H 21–24 months

For each of the following teeth, choose the most appropriate eruption dates from the list above. You may use each option once, more than once or not at all.

1 Lower right A.
2 Upper right C.
3 Lower left D.

1.8 Theme: Dates of Eruption (2)

A	4-5 years	G	10-11 years
B	5-6 years	H	11-12 years
C	6-7 years	I	12-13 years
D	7-8 years	J	13-14 years
E	8-9 years	K	14-15 years
F	9-10 years	L	15-16 years

For each of the following teeth, choose the most appropriate eruption date from the list above. You may use each option once, more than once or not at all.

1 Maxillary first permanent premolar
2 Maxillary first permanent molar
3 Mandibular second premolar
4 Mandibular first permanent molar
5 Mandibular second permanent molar

1.9 Theme: Dates of Eruption (3)

A	1-2 months	G	12-15 months
B	2-3 months	H	15-18 months
C	4-5 months	I	18-21 months
D	6-7 months	J	21-24 months
E	7-8 months	K	24-36 months
F	9-10 months	L	36-48 months

For each of the following teeth, choose the most appropriate eruption date from the list above. You may use each option once, more than once or not at all.

1 Maxillary deciduous central incisor
2 Mandibular deciduous lower canine
3 Maxillary deciduous lateral incisor
4 Mandibular deciduous first molar
5 Maxillary deciduous second molar

CHILD DENTAL HEALTH AND ORTHODONTICS

1.10 Theme: Dental Trauma (1)

A   Ankylosis
B   Autotransplantation
C   Avulsion
D   Concussion
E   Extrusion
F   Implantation
G   Intrusion
H   Luxation
I   Reimplantation
J   Subluxation
K   Transplantation

For each of the following statements, choose the most appropriate term from the list above. You may use each option once, more than once or not at all.

1   The loss of a tooth from its socket, which is then replaced in the same socket.
2   The removal of a tooth from its socket, which is then placed in another position within the mouth.
3   The loosening of a tooth within its socket without any displacement.
4   Injury to the supporting tissues without any displacement of the tooth.
5   The displacement of a tooth into its socket.

1.11 Theme: Dental Trauma (2)

A   3 days
B   1 week
C   1–2 weeks
D   2–3 weeks
E   3–5 weeks
F   6–9 weeks
G   9–12 weeks
H   12–16 weeks
I   6 months
J   1 year
K   2 years
L   Do not splint

For each of the following injuries, choose the correct length of splinting time required from the list above. You may use each option once, more than once or not at all.

1   Extrusion of a maxillary permanent central incisor.
2   Avulsion of a maxillary deciduous central incisor.
3   Luxation of a mandibular permanent canine.
4   Subluxation of a mandibular permanent lateral incisor with associated alveolar bone fracture, but no comminution.
5   A middle third root fracture of a maxillary permanent central incisor.

1.12 Theme: Behaviour Management

A Association
B Behaviour shaping
C Desensitisation
D Disassociation
E Modelling
F Reinforcement
G Sensitisation
H Show, tell, do
I Tell, show, do

For each of the following statements, choose the most appropriate term from the list above. You may use each option once, more than once or not at all.

1 The process of influencing behaviour towards a desired ideal.

2 Describing the treatment which is going to be performed, then visually demonstrating it, followed by performing the treatment on the child.

3 The strengthening of a pattern of behaviour which increases the probability that the behaviour will be displayed in the future.

4 A three-stage process: first, training the patient to relax; second, constructing a hierarchy of fear-producing stimuli related to the patient's principal fear; and third, introducing the stimulus in the relaxed patient until it causes no fear.

5 Letting a child watch another child have dental treatment to show that there is nothing for them to fear.

CHILD DENTAL HEALTH AND ORTHODONTICS

1.13 Theme: Tooth Size

A	5 mm	G	8.5 mm
B	6 mm	H	9 mm
C	6.5 mm	I	10 mm
D	7 mm	J	11 mm
E	7.5 mm	K	12 mm
F	8 mm	L	13 mm

For each of the following teeth, choose the correct mesiodistal width from the list above. You may use each option once, more than once or not at all.

1. Maxillary permanent central incisor.
2. Maxillary permanent first premolar.
3. Maxillary permanent second premolar.
4. Mandibular permanent lateral incisor.
5. Mandibular permanent first molar.

1.14 Theme: Cephalometrics (1)

A	Anterior nasal spine	I	Menton
B	Articulare	J	Nasion
C	Frankfort plane	K	Oribitale
D	Glabella	L	Point A
E	Gnathion	M	Point B
F	Gonion	N	Porion
G	Mandibular plane	O	Sella
H	Maxillary plane		

For each of the following cephalometric points/planes, choose the most appropriate anatomical name from the list above. You may use each option once, more than once or not at all.

1. The most prominent point over the frontal bone.
2. The most anterior and inferior point on the bony chin.
3. The plane through the anterior nasal spine and the posterior nasal spine.
4. The mid-point of the sella turcica.
5. The deepest point on the mandibular profile between pogonion and the alveolar crest.

1.15 Theme: Cephalometrics (2)

A	Anterior nasal spine		I	Menton
B	Articulare		J	Nasion
C	Frankfort plane		K	Oribitale
D	Glabella		L	Point A
E	Gnathion		M	Point B
F	Gonion		N	Porion
G	Mandibular plane		O	Sella
H	Maxillary plane			

For each of the following cephalometric planes/points, choose the most appropriate anatomical name from the list above. You may use each option once, more than once or not at all.

1. The projection on a lateral skull radiograph of the posterior outline of the condylar process on the inferior outline of the cranial base.
2. The most posterior and inferior point at the angle of the mandible.
3. The plane through menton which forms a tangent to the inferior border of the angle of the mandible.
4. The plane passing through orbitale and porion.
5. The uppermost point on the external acoustic meatus.

1.16 Theme: Occlusion (1)

A	Anterior oral seal		F	Malocclusion
B	Centric occlusion		G	Normal occlusion
C	Competent lips		H	Occlusion
D	Dental arch		I	Posterior oral seal
E	Incompetent lips			

For each of the following statements, choose the most appropriate term from the list above. You may use each option once, more than once or not at all.

1. The curved contour of the dentition or the residual ridge.
2. When, with the mandible in rest position, muscular effort is required to obtain lip seal.
3. A seal produced by contact between the lips or between tongue and lower lip.
4. The position of maximum intercuspation, which is also the position of centric relation.
5. A seal between the dorsum of the tongue and the soft palate.

1.17 Theme: Occlusion (2)

A   Complete overbite
B   Complete overjet
C   Ideal occlusion
D   Incomplete overbite
E   Incomplete overjet
F   Malocclusion
G   Normal occlusion
H   Overbite
I   Overjet

For each of the following statements, choose the most appropriate term from the list above. You may use each option once, more than once or not at all.

1. An occlusion which satisfies the requirement of function and aesthetics but in which there are minor irregularities of individual teeth.
2. The relation between upper and lower incisors in the horizontal plane.
3. The overlap of the lower incisors by the upper incisors in the vertical plane.
4. An overbite in which the lower incisors make contact with either the upper incisors or the palate.
5. An overbite in which the lower incisors contact neither the upper incisors nor the palatal mucosa.

1.18 Theme: Terminology

A Buccal segments
B Cingulum plateau
C Crossbite
D Diastema
E Incisor angulation
F Incisor inclination
G Labial segments
H Leeway space
I Primate space

For each of the following statements, choose the most appropriate term from the list above. You may use each option once, more than once or not at all.

1 The incisor teeth as a whole.
2 A naturally occurring space in the deciduous dentition, mesial to the upper canine and distal to the lower canine.
3 The extra space provided for the permanent dentition when the deciduous canines and molars are replaced by the permanent canines and premolars.
4 An expression of tip in the labiopalatal plane.
5 An expression of tip in the mesiodistal plane.

1.19 Theme: Dental Anomalies

A Anodontia
B Cingulum pit
C Dens in dente
D Dilaceration
E Macrodontia
F Microdontia
G Odontome
H Oligodontia
I Palatal invaginatus
J Polydontia
K Supernumerary teeth
L Supplemental teeth

For each of the following descriptions of dental anomalies, choose the most appropriate name from the list above. You may use each option once, more than once or not at all.

1 An enamel-lined invagination sometimes present on the palatal surface of upper incisors.
2 Abnormally small teeth, often the last of a series.
3 The developmental absence of a number of teeth.
4 Teeth in excess of the usual number – usually of abnormal form.
5 Supernumerary teeth resembling normal teeth.

CHILD DENTAL HEALTH AND ORTHODONTICS

1.20 Theme: Index of Orthodontic Treatment Needs (IOTN)

A	0	E	4
B	1	F	5
C	2	G	6
D	3	H	7

For each of the following scenarios, choose the most appropriate IOTN category from the list above. You may use each option once, more than once or not at all.

1. Increased overjet greater than 9 mm.
2. Extremely minor malocclusions, including minor contact point displacements less than 1 mm.
3. Reverse overjet greater than 1 mm but less than 3.5 mm with incompetent lips.
4. Increased and complete overbite with gingival or palatal trauma.
5. Point contact displacements greater than 1 mm but less than or equal to 2 mm.

1.21 Theme: Fluoride

A 0.1 mg fluoride/day
B 0.25 mg fluoride/day
C 0.5 mg fluoride/day
D 0.75 mg fluoride/day
E 1.0 mg fluoride/day
F 2.0 mg fluoride/day
G 5.0 mg fluoride/day
H No fluoride required

For each of the following scenarios, choose the most appropriate dosage of fluoride from the list above. You may use each option once, more than once or not at all.

1. A 3-month-old child living in an area with water fluoridation greater than 0.7 ppm.
2. A 5-year-old child living in an area with no water fluoridation.
3. A 3-year-old child living in an area with water fluoridation of 0.2 ppm.
4. An 18-month-old child living in an area with water fluoridation of 0.25 ppm.
5. A 3-year-old child living in an area with water fluoridation of 0.6 ppm.

1.22 Theme: Tooth-brushing Techniques (2)

A Bass
B Charter's
C Fones
D Modified Stillman
E Roll
F Scrub
G Stillman

For each of the following brushing techniques, choose the most appropriate name from the list above. You may use each option once, more than once or not at all.

1. Pointing the brush apically, parallel to the long axis of the teeth, roll the brush occlusally maintaining contact with the gingivae, then with the tooth surface.

2. Pointing the brush apically, at 45° to the long axis of the teeth, vibrate the brush, not changing the position of the bristles.

3. Pointing the brush apically, at 45° to the long axis of the teeth, apply pressure to blanch the gingivae. Repeat several times. Slightly rotate the brush occlusally during the procedure.

4. Pointing the brush apically, at 45° to the long axis of the teeth, make the gingivae blanch, but at the same time vibrate the brush and move it occlusally.

5. Pointing the brush horizontally with the teeth in occlusion, move the brush in a rotary motion against the maxillary and mandibular teeth surfaces and gingival margins.

1.23 Theme: Cephalometrics (3)

A 3 ± 2°
B 27 ± 4°
C 79 ± 3°
D 81 ± 3°
E 133 ± 10°

For each of the following angles traced on a cephalogram, choose the most appropriate value from the list above. You may use each option once, more than once or not at all.

1. SNA
2. SNB
3. ANB
4. MMPA
5. Interincisal angle

1.24 Theme: Skeletal Relationships, Mandibular Positions and Paths of Closure

A	Alveolar process
B	Bimaxillary
C	Deviation of the mandible
D	Displacement of the mandible
E	Freeway space
F	Habit position
G	Intermaxillary space
H	Premature contact
I	Proclination
J	Prognathism
K	Rest position
L	Skeletal bases
M	Skeletal pattern

For each of the following descriptions, choose the most appropriate term from the list above. You may use each option once, more than once or not at all.

1. The parts of the mandible and maxilla whose development and presence depends on the teeth.
2. The maxilla and the mandible, excluding the alveolar processes.
3. The relation between the mandible and maxilla in the antero-posterior axis.
4. The space between the upper and lower skeletal bases when the mandible is in the rest position.
5. The excessive projection of a jaw from beneath the cranial base.
6. Pertaining to both jaws.
7. The labial tipping of incisor teeth, often together with the supporting alveolar process.
8. The position of the mandible in which the muscles acting on it show little activity.
9. The interocclusal clearance when the mandible is in the rest position.
10. A sagittal movement of the mandible during closure from a position of centric occlusion.

1.25 Theme: Treatment of Deciduous Teeth

A Extraction under general anaesthetic
B Extraction under local anaesthetic
C Fissure sealants only
D Non-vital pulpotomy
E No treatment required
F Preventive and dietary advice only
G Simple restoration
H Simple restoration and fissure sealants
I Systemic fluoride only
J Topical fluoride and preventive advice
K Vital pulpotomy

For each of the following scenarios, choose the most appropriate treatment from the list above. You may use each option once, more than once or not at all.

1 A 6-year-old child with a small carious lesion in a lower right second molar. He is cooperative and his first permanent molars have erupted.

2 A 4-year-old child with six first and second molars that cannot be restored.

3 A 2-year-old child with a single tiny pit caries lesion in an upper first molar.

4 A 5-year-old child who has caries in his lower left first molar which is causing the tooth to throb. The tooth is vital.

5 A 7-year-old child with a non-vital lower left second molar.

CHILD DENTAL HEALTH AND ORTHODONTICS

1.26 Theme: Dates of Calcification

A	Birth	H	15-18 months
B	1-2 months	I	18-21 months
C	2-3 months	J	21-24 months
D	3-4 months	K	24-30 months
E	4-5 months	L	30-36 months
F	6-7 months	M	36-42 months
G	12-15 months		

For each of the following teeth, choose the most appropriate calcification date from the list above. You may use each option once, more than once or not at all.

1. Mandibular second permanent molars
2. Mandibular first permanent molars
3. Maxillary central incisors
4. Maxillary canines
5. Maxillary first premolars

1.27 Theme: Malocclusion

A   Class I
B   Class II division 1
C   Class II division 2
D   Class III

For each of the following findings, choose the most appropriate diagnosis of malocclusion from the list above. You may use each option once, more than once or not at all.

1. The lower anteriors lie anterior to the cingulum plateau of the upper incisors.
2. The lower arch is at least one half cusp width post-normal to the upper and the upper central incisors and lateral incisors are retroclined.
3. The lower arch is at least one half cusp width post-normal to the upper and the upper central incisors are retroclined, but the lateral incisors are proclined.
4. The lower incisor edges lie posterior to the cingulum plateau of the upper incisors and there is an increased overjet.
5. The lower incisor edges occlude with or lie directly below the cingulum plateau of the upper incisors.

18 CHILD DENTAL HEALTH AND ORTHODONTICS

1.28 Theme: General Paediatric Conditions

A   Asthma
B   Duodenal atresia
C   Eczema
D   Epilepsy
E   Hand foot and mouth
F   Herpetic gingivostomatitis
G   Impetigo
H   Measles
I   Mumps
J   Pneumonia
K   Trigeminal neuralgia

For each of the following medications, choose the most appropriate condition from the list above. You may use each option once, more than once or not at all.

1   Sodium valproate
2   Aciclovir
3   Flucloxacillin
4   Hydrocortisone
5   Salbutamol

1.29 Theme: Dates of Eruption and Chronological Age

A   0 month
B   2 months
C   4 months
D   6 months
E   6-7 years
F   7-8 years
G   8-9 years
H   9-10 years
I   10-11 years
J   11-12 years
K   12-13 years
L   13-14 years
M   14-15 years

For each of the following children, choose the most appropriate chronological age from the list above. You may use each option once, more than once or not at all.

1   A child has all teeth fully erupted, except her second permanent molars which are partially erupted.
2   A child has her very first deciduous teeth erupting.
3   The maxillary permanent canines are erupting.
4   The mandibular permanent canines are erupting.
5   The mandibular permanent lateral incisors are erupting.

CHILD DENTAL HEALTH AND ORTHODONTICS

1.30 Theme: Abnormalities of Eruption

A Abnormal position of tooth crypt
B Congenital absence
C Dilaceration
D Early loss of deciduous predecessor
E Primary failure of eruption
F Retention of deciduous tooth
G Supernumerary tooth

For each of the following problems, choose the most likely cause from the list above. You may use each option once, more than once or not at all.

1 Failure of upper lateral incisor to appear.
2 Crowding.
3 Failure of eruption of upper central incisor.
4 Palatal position of upper canine.
5 Delayed eruption of lower first permanent molar.

1.31 Theme: Abnormalities of Tooth Structure/Number

A Amelogenesis imperfecta
B Amoxicillin
C Cleidocranial dysostosis
D Dentinogenesis imperfecta
E Down syndrome
F Ectodermal dysplasia
G Hydrocortisone
H Kernicterus
I Local infection
J Paget's disease
K Tetracycline

For each of the following statements, choose the most appropriate diagnosis from the list above. You may use each option once, more than once or not at all.

1 Anodontia.
2 Exaggerated transverse diameter of cranium; delayed fontanelle closure; hypoplastic teeth; hypomineralisation; hypoplastic clavicles.
3 Single tooth with brown hypoplastic crown (Turner tooth).
4 All teeth hypoplastic, enamel is brown-yellow, teeth are soft and chip under attrition.
5 Yellow, brown or green hyperpigmentation of teeth. Child had recurrent ear and chest infections.

1.1 Child Development

1	F	18 months
2	H	36 months
3	B	4 months
4	C	6 months
5	D	9 months

It is important for health care workers to recognise a normally developing child. Children do not have the dexterity to brush their own teeth until they are able to write well, which is normally 7 years old, hence parents should brush a child's teeth. Normally developing infants can only drink from a cup at about 12 months, and dentists should give appropriate advice about avoiding sugary drinks in bottles at night for infants. Walking independently usually occurs at 15 months and running at 24 months. At five years a child should be able to tie their own shoe laces. Lack of skills especially in older children may also be due to parental neglect.

1.2 Childhood Illnesses

1	E	Polio
2	F	Rubella
3	G	Tuberculosis
4	D	Pertussis
5	C	Mumps

Diphtheria may start with a sore throat, fever and a characteristic cough. Complications may include myocarditis and death in 5-10% of cases.

Initial manifestations of *Haemophilus meningitis*, seen in more than half of all cases of *Haemophilus influenzae* type b (Hib) meningitis, include altered cry, change in mentation, nausea or vomiting, fever, headache, photophobia, irritability, anorexia and seizures.

CHILD DENTAL HEALTH AND ORTHODONTICS

Pertussis is also known as 'whooping cough'.

Polio or infantile paralysis is spread from person to person by oral faecal route. Oral vaccination is effective in preventing this serious disease.

Tuberculosis is on the rise again in the UK and western countries; the BCG (Bacillus Calmette-Guérin) vaccination offers protection in 8 out of 10 individuals. Heaf and Mantoux tests may be used to check immunity.

Rubella or German measles causes a pink-red rash with high temperature. The consequences are serious if a pregnant woman develops symptoms, with the fetus at risk of deafness, cataracts and heart defects, also known as congenital rubella syndrome (CRS). The MMR (measles, mumps and rubella) vaccine has reduced the incidence of CRS.

Varicella zoster causes chicken pox in children – a mild, common childhood illness with a characteristic rash.

1.3 Chromosomal Abnormalities

| 1 | D | Trisomy 21 |

| 2 | C | Trisomy 18 |

| 3 | B | Trisomy 13 |

| 4 | A | 45 XO |

Down syndrome is typically associated with physical growth delays, characteristic facial features, and mild-to-moderate intellectual disability.

The majority of fetuses with Edward syndrome die before birth.

A high number of fetuses with Patau syndrome do not survive birth; those that do often have microcephaly, spinal and ocular defects.

Turner syndrome affects only females; they often have a short webbed neck, low set ears, small in stature but normal intelligence.

Individuals with Pierre Robin syndrome have facial malformations, cleft palate, retrognathia and glossoptosis. Pierre Robin sequence may be caused by genetic anomalies at chromosome 2.

Dentists are sometimes the first health care workers to recognise individuals with syndromes from their dental and facial characteristics.

CHILD DENTAL HEALTH AND ORTHODONTICS

1.4 International Caries Detection and Assessment System (ICDAS-II codes)

1 F 5

2 C 2

3 G 6

4 B 1

5 E 4

ICDAS is a simple caries detection and assessment system for clinical practice, dental education and research.

International Caries Detection and Assessment System (ICDAS-II)

Code	Criteria
0	Sound tooth surface after prolonged air drying (more than 5 seconds)
1	First visual change in enamel after prolonged air drying (more than 5 seconds)
2	Distinct visual change in enamel seen when wet
3	Localised enamel breakdown seen when wet but no signs of dentine involvement
4	Underlying dark shadow from dentine
5	Distinct cavity with visible dentine
6	Extensive (more than half of surface) distinct cavity with visible dentine

1.5 Trauma to the Primary Dentition

1 H Root fracture

An apical third root fracture has occurred. The trauma has caused the coronal two-thirds to separate, resulting in the supra-occlusion. If the tooth is only minimally displaced and relatively firm, it may be kept under review and may exfoliate as normal. However, if the coronal fragment is loose, extract this and leave the apical fragment to be resorbed with eruption of the secondary dentition

2 F Intrusive luxation

Intrusive luxation is a common injury for toddlers who are learning to walk. If the teeth are firm and not displaced into the developing tooth germ, spontaneous re-eruption usually occurs. If it does not re-erupt, then ankylosis is likely and extraction may be necessary to prevent ectopic eruption of the secondary successor.

3 C Crown fracture

A crown fracture has occurred. If only enamel and dentine are involved, it is considered uncomplicated; however, if the pulp is involved, it is considered a complicated fracture. Uncomplicated crown fractures can generally be restored and monitored. If complicated by pulpal involvement, pulp capping or pulpotomy may be considered, depending upon the size of the pulpal exposure and length of time before treatment has been sought.

4 B Concussion

This is a concussion injury, as the tooth is tender but there is no increase in mobility.

5 E Extrusive luxation

Extrusive luxation usually results in greater mobility and spontaneous alignment may occur in minor displacements. However, if seen early after the trauma, gentle repositioning may be possible with finger pressure. If seen late after the trauma, extraction may be considered.

1.6 Tooth-brushing Techniques (1)

1	E	Vibrate the brush while moving it apically into the gingival margin
2	D	Vibrate the brush, not changing the position of the bristles
3	A	Apply pressure to blanch the gingivae, then remove. Repeat several times. Slightly rotate the brush and gradually move it occlusally

The most accepted method is the Bass technique.

The Bass method: Position the toothbrush

- Direct the nylon filaments apically (up for maxillary, down for mandibular teeth) at a 45° angle. It is usually easier and safer if you first place the brush parallel with the long axis of the tooth.
- From that position the brush can be turned slightly and brought down to the gingival margin to the 45° angle.

The Bass method: Angle the filaments at gum–tooth margin

- Place the toothbrush with the flat brushing plane and rounded nylon filament tips directed straight into the gingival sulcus or gingival margin.
- The filaments will be directed at approximately 45° to the long axis of the tooth.

The Bass method: Strokes

- Press lightly without flexing and bending the filaments.
- Nylon filament tips will enter the gingival sulci at gum–tooth border and cover the gum margin.
- Vibrate the toothbrush back and forth with very short strokes without disengaging the nylon tips of the filaments from the gum margin. Count at least 10 vibrations.
- Reposition the toothbrush and apply the brush to the next group of two or three teeth. Take care to overlap placement.
- Repeat the entire stroke at each position around the maxillary and mandibular arches, for both facial and lingual surfaces.

1.7 Dates of Eruption (1)

1   C   6–9 months

2   G   18–21 months

3   E   12–15 months

Tooth	Eruption dates (months)
Deciduous incisors	6–9
Deciduous canines	18–21
Deciduous first molars	12–15
Deciduous second molars	24–36

1.8 Dates of Eruption (2)

1   G   10–11 years

2   C   6–7 years

3   H   11–12 years

4   B   5–6 years

5   I   12–13 years

It is important to know the normal eruption dates so that you can recognise what is abnormal and when to investigate for missing teeth.

Tooth	Eruption dates (years)
Mandibular first permanent molar	5–6
Maxillary first permanent molar	6–7
Maxillary first permanent premolar	10–11
Mandibular second permanent premolar	11–12
Mandibular second permanent molar	12–13

1.9 Dates of Eruption (3)

1 D 6-7 months

2 H 15-18 months

3 E 7-8 months

4 G 12-15 months

5 K 24-36 months

It is important to know the normal eruption dates so that you can recognise what is abnormal and when to investigate for missing teeth.

Tooth	Eruption dates (months)
Maxillary deciduous central incisor	6-7
Maxillary deciduous lateral incisor	7-8
Mandibular deciduous first molar	12-15
Mandibular deciduous lower canine	15-18
Maxillary deciduous second molar	24-36

1.10 Dental Trauma (1)

1 I Reimplantation

2 K Transplantation

3 J Subluxation

4 D Concussion

5 G Intrusion

You should be able to describe and recognise traumatic injuries to teeth, as different injuries require vastly different treatments.

1.11 Dental Trauma (2)

1	C	1-2 weeks
2	L	Do not splint
3	D	2-3 weeks
4	E	3-5 weeks
5	G	9-12 weeks

Teeth should not be splinted for more than three months as the risk of ankylosis increases. An extruded tooth should be replaced in the correct anatomical position using digital pressure under local anaesthetic. Deciduous teeth should not be reimplanted, and therefore they do not require splinting. If a subluxed tooth is not mobile, then splinting is not required but if it is mobile and there is an associated alveolar bone fracture, then 3-5 weeks of splinting is required.

1.12 Behaviour Management

1	B	Behaviour shaping
2	I	Tell, show, do
3	F	Reinforcement
4	C	Desensitisation
5	E	Modelling

Behaviour shaping is based on the planned introduction of treatment procedures, so that the child is gradually trained to accept treatment in a relaxed and cooperative manner. Start with examination, then topical fluoride application, then a minimal restoration, and then until local anaesthetic is accepted. Reinforcement is using plenty of encouragement for positive behaviour from the child, e.g. the dentist tells the child 'well done' and rewards the child with a treat after treatment.

1.13 Tooth Size

1 G 8.5 mm

2 D 7 mm

3 C 6.5 mm

4 B 6 mm

5 J 11 mm

Knowing the different widths of teeth helps you work out the space that will be available after planned orthodontic extractions.

CHILD DENTAL HEALTH AND ORTHODONTICS

1.14 Cephalometrics (1)

| 1 | D | Glabella |

| 2 | E | Gnathion |

| 3 | H | Maxillary plane |

(ANS + PNS on diagram below)

| 4 | O | Sella |

| 5 | M | Point B |

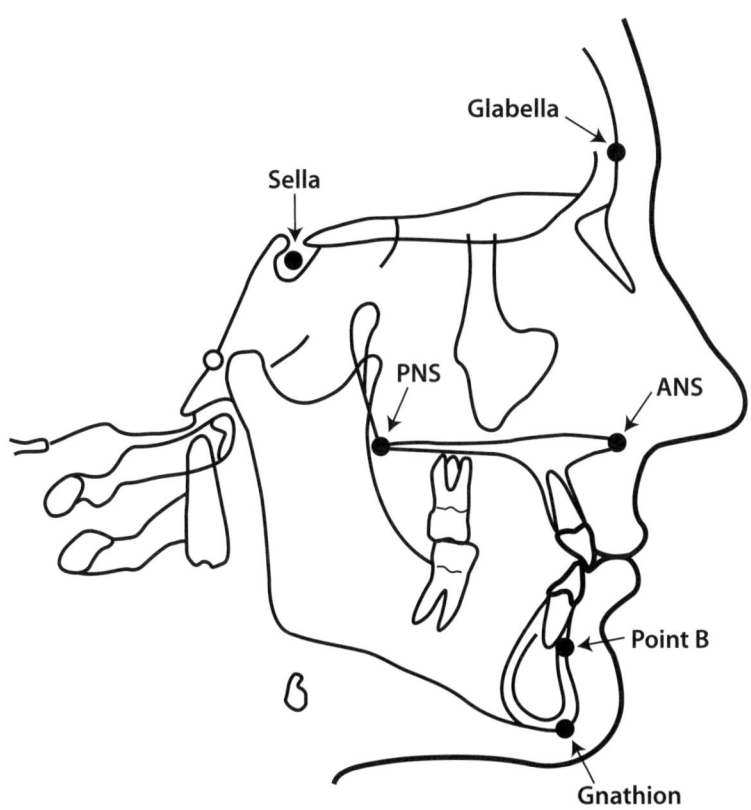

CHILD DENTAL HEALTH AND ORTHODONTICS

1.15 Cephalometrics (2)

1 B Articulare

2 F Gonion

3 G Mandibular plane

4 C Frankfort plane

5 N Porion

Knowledge of the correct points and planes on a lateral cephalogram helps correlation of the physical findings in a patient with the radiographic findings. You should know the definitions of the various anatomical points on the face to be able to find them on the cephalogram.

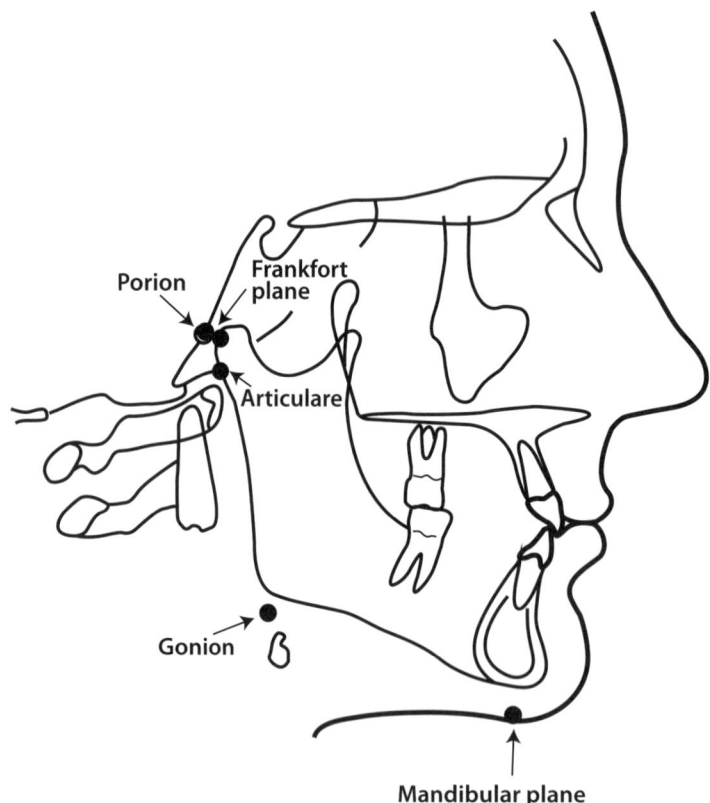

CHILD DENTAL HEALTH AND ORTHODONTICS

1.16 Occlusion (1)

1	D	Dental arch
2	E	Incompetent lips
3	A	Anterior oral seal
4	B	Centric occlusion
5	I	Posterior oral seal

There is a lot of jargon in orthodontics and when describing a patient it is important to use the correct terminology.

1.17 Occlusion (2)

1	G	Normal occlusion
2	I	Overjet
3	H	Overbite
4	A	Complete overbite
5	D	Incomplete overbite

The above terminology is used when describing malocclusions, and some need to be measured, e.g. overjet and overbite.

CHILD DENTAL HEALTH AND ORTHODONTICS

1.18 Terminology

1 G Labial segments

2 I Primate space

3 H Leeway space

4 F Incisor inclination

5 E Incisor angulation

As stated before, knowledge of orthodontic jargon is useful when explaining or describing occlusion of patients.

1.19 Dental Anomalies

1 C Dens in dente

2 F Microdontia

3 H Oligodontia

4 K Supernumerary teeth

5 L Supplemental teeth

Dental anomalies should be recognised and described in patients. This topic is further covered in Chapter 4.

CHILD DENTAL HEALTH AND ORTHODONTICS

1.20 IOTN

1 F 5

2 B 1

3 D 3

4 F 5

5 C 2

The IOTN classification is from 1 to 5, where 1 is 'no treatment is required' and 5 is 'severe malocclusion and treatment is required'.

1.21 Fluoride

1 H No fluoride required

2 E 1.0 mg fluoride/day

3 C 0.5 mg fluoride/day

4 B 0.25 mg fluoride/day

5 B 0.25 mg fluoride/day

Children younger than 6 months of age should not be given fluoride supplements, regardless of the level of water fluoridation. Between 6 months and 2 years of age the child should have supplementation only if there is less than 0.3 ppm of fluoride in the water. In this case the dosage should be 0.25 mg fluoride/day. Between 2 and 4 years of age the dose should be 0.5 mg fluoride/day in areas with water fluoridation of less than 0.3 ppm and 0.25 mg fluoride/day where it is between 0.3 and 0.7 ppm. Over 4 years of age the dose should be 1.0 mg fluoride/day in areas with water fluoridation of less than 0.3 ppm and 0.5 mg fluoride/day where water fluoridation is between 0.3 and 0.7 ppm.

CHILD DENTAL HEALTH AND ORTHODONTICS

1.22 Tooth-brushing Techniques (2)

1 E Roll

2 A Bass

3 G Stillman

4 D Modified Stillman

5 C Fones

Oral hygiene instruction is a very important part of paediatric dentistry. Preventive advice is often more valuable than the physical treatment provided. A good brushing technique is important, so that all teeth are cleaned properly and not harmed by an incorrect technique.

1.23 Cephalometrics (3)

1 D 81 ± 3°

2 C 79 ± 3°

3 A 3 ± 2°

4 B 27 ± 4°

5 E 133 ± 10°

Cephalometric measurements are very important when diagnosing skeletal relationships, and the above angles (and the ranges) describe the normal skeletal relationship.

CHILD DENTAL HEALTH AND ORTHODONTICS

1.24 Skeletal Relationships, Mandibular Positions and Paths of Closure

1   A   Alveolar process

2   L   Skeletal bases

3   M   Skeletal pattern

4   G   Intermaxillary space

5   J   Prognathism

6   B   Bimaxillary

7   I   Proclination

8   K   Rest position

9   E   Freeway space

10 D   Displacement of the mandible

The above definitions should be learnt so that you can describe a patient and their occlusion/malocclusion adequately.

CHILD DENTAL HEALTH AND ORTHODONTICS

1.25 Treatment of Deciduous Teeth

1 H Simple restoration and fissure sealants

2 A Extraction under general anaesthetic

3 J Topical fluoride and preventive advice

4 K Vital pulpotomy

5 G Simple restoration

Dentistry can be very subjective, however the above scenarios are quite realistic and definitive. It is unrealistic that a 4-year-old child would be able to cope with six extractions under local anaesthetic, so a general anaesthetic is more likely in this scenario.

1.26 Dates of Calcification

1 L 30-36 months

2 A Birth

3 D 3-4 months

4 E 4-5 months

5 I 18-21 months

Calcification dates should be learned – this knowledge can be applied in many areas, ranging from fluoride prescription to estimation of a child's age from a radiograph.

Tooth	Calcification dates (months)
First molars	Birth
Maxillary central incisors	3-4
Maxillary central and mandibular lateral incisors	3-4
Maxillary lateral incisors	10-12
Mandibular canines	4-5
Maxillary first premolars	18-21
Mandibular first premolars	21-24
Maxillary second premolars	24-27
Maxillary canines	4-5
Mandibular second premolars	27-30
Second molars	30-36
Third molars	80-120

1.27 Malocclusion

1 D Class III

2 C Class II division 2

3 C Class II division 2

4 C Class II division 2

5 A Class I

The relationship of the central incisors is important when describing the classification of the labial segments. The trick question is Q 3, where you must decide on the basis of the relationship of the central incisors and disregard the positioning of the lateral incisors.

CHILD DENTAL HEALTH AND ORTHODONTICS

1.28 General Paediatric Conditions

1 D Epilepsy

2 F Herpetic gingivostomatitis

3 G Impetigo

4 C Eczema

5 A Asthma

Epilepsy in children is commonly treated with sodium valproate. Aciclovir can be used in herpes, but the majority of cases can usually be managed with fluids, analgesia and reassurance. Flucloxacillin is used to treat impetigo, a common bacterial infection. Pneumonia in children is either viral or responds well to amoxicillin. Eczema is treated with hydrocortisone, emollients and antihistamines to reduce the itchiness. Asthma is treated with salbutamol, betamethasone and if severe, oral steroids.

1.29 Dates of Eruption and Chronological Age

1 K 12-13 years

2 D 6 months

3 J 11-12 years

4 H 9-10 years

5 F 7-8 years

The above scenarios apply the knowledge gained from previous questions indirectly, and should gauge what has been learnt so far in this chapter.

CHILD DENTAL HEALTH AND ORTHODONTICS

1.30 Abnormalities of Eruption

1	B	Congenital absence
2	D	Early loss of deciduous predecessor
3	G	Supernumerary tooth
4	A	Abnormal position of tooth crypt
5	E	Primary failure of eruption

Absence of teeth and delayed eruption of permanent teeth are common problems in children and a good knowledge of the reasons why this happens is required.

1.31 Abnormalities of Tooth Structure/Number

1	F	Ectodermal dysplasia
2	C	Cleidocranial dysostosis
3	I	Local infection
4	A	Amelogenesis imperfecta
5	K	Tetracycline

Anodontia is classically caused by ectodermal dysplasia, and the patient also has absent sweat glands. Q 4 describes amelogenesis imperfecta rather than dentinogenesis imperfecta where the enamel is more or less normal but chips off because the bond to the dentine is weak. Tetracycline is the classic cause of drug-induced intrinsic staining. The hint in the question is that the child has had recurrent chest and ear infections.

2 General Medicine

2.1 Theme: Eating Disorders
2.2 Theme: HIV/AIDS
2.3 Theme: UK Malignancy death rate
2.4 Theme: Personality Disorders
2.5 Theme: Shortness of Breath in Children
2.6 Theme: Vitamin Deficiency
2.7 Theme: Complications of Myocardial Infarction
2.8 Theme: Glasgow Coma Scale Score
2.9 Theme: Cardiovascular Examination Findings
2.10 Theme: Renal Disease
2.11 Theme: Endocrine Disease
2.12 Theme: Examination of the Head and Neck
2.13 Theme: Weight Loss
2.14 Theme: Lung Disorders
2.15 Theme: Back Pain
2.16 Theme: Abdominal Masses
2.17 Theme: Diabetic Complications
2.18 Theme: Liver
2.19 Theme: Lymphadenopathy
2.20 Theme: Abdominal Distension
2.21 Theme: Loss of Consciousness
2.22 Theme: Chest Pain
2.23 Theme: Eye Disease
2.24 Theme: Abdominal Pain
2.25 Theme: Collapse
2.26 Theme: Hand Signs
2.27 Theme: General Conditions
2.28 Theme: Diarrhoea and Vomiting
2.29 Theme: Respiratory Diagnosis
2.30 Theme: Infections
2.31 Theme: Endocrine Conditions
2.32 Theme: Severe Infections
2.33 Theme: Lower-limb Problems
2.34 Theme: Pre-operative Investigations
2.35 Theme: Infections of the Lung
2.36 Theme: Tests

2.1 Theme: Eating Disorders

A   Achalasia
B   Anorexia
C   Bulimia
D   Myasthenia gravis
E   Oesophageal candidiasis
F   Pharyngeal pouch
G   Plummer–Vinson syndrome
H   Reflux oesophagitis

For each of the following scenarios, choose the most appropriate diagnosis from the list above. You may use each option once, more than once or not at all.

1   A 21-year-old female who is of normal weight, complains of thin and chipped incisors which are sharp and sensitive.

2   A 45-year-old female who is obese complains of 'heart burn' after eating and lying down. She has noticed excessive salivation and wheezing when supine.

3   A 47-year-old female complains of food sticking in the back of the throat. She exhibits spoon-shaped nails and has a smooth tongue.

4   A 65-year-old male complains of difficulty in swallowing, especially after the first mouthful, unless he regurgitates. A neck swelling is evident.

5   A 31-year-old female presents for dental treatment. She is very underweight but considers that she needs to lose more weight.

GENERAL MEDICINE

2.2 Theme: HIV/AIDS

A   *Candida albicans*
B   *Cryptococcus*
C   Cytomegalovirus (CMV)
D   Epstein–Barr virus (EBV)
E   Human herpesvirus 8
F   *Streptococcus*
G   *Toxoplasma gondii*

From the options listed above, choose the one which can lead to the following conditions for patients with HIV/AIDS. You may use each option once, more than once or not at all.

1   Intracerebral lymphoma
2   Kaposi's sarcoma
3   Odynophagia
4   Retinitis
5   The most common type of pneumonia

2.3 Theme: UK Malignancy Death Rate

A   5000
B   10 000
C   15 000
D   20 000
E   25 000
F   30 000
G   35 000
H   40 000

For the following organs affected by malignancy, choose the closest death rate per annum from the options above. You may use each option once, more than once or not at all.

1   Breast
2   Colorectal
3   Lung
4   Lymphoma
5   Pancreas
6   Prostate

GENERAL MEDICINE

2.4 Theme: Personality Disorders

A	Affective	E	Histrionic
B	Anxious	F	Narcissism
C	Borderline	G	Obsessive-compulsive
D	Dependent	H	Schizoid

For each of the following descriptions, choose the most appropriate personality disorder from the list above. You may use each option once, more than once or not at all.

1. Abnormal sense of self-importance, ideas of success, power and intellectual superiority.
2. Emotionally detached and cold, self-sufficient, introspective with potential to fantasise.
3. Unstable relationships, impulsivity, variable moods and chronic feelings of emptiness.
4. Unduly compliant, lack vigour and self-reliance. Avoid responsibility.
5. Unduly focused on unimportant detail and resultant indecision.

2.5 Theme: Shortness of Breath in Children

A	Acute asthma
B	Croup
C	Heart failure
D	Inhaled foreign body
E	Pneumonia
F	Tuberculosis
G	Whooping cough

For each of the clinical scenarios below, choose the most likely diagnosis from the list above. Each option maybe used once, more than once or not at all.

1. A 2-year-old boy who develops a barking cough with stridor.
2. A 3-year-old girl with unilateral wheeze and shortness of breath.
3. A 5-year-old boy with a long-term chronic cough which develops into gasping for breath with a characteristic noise.
4. A 12-year-old boy with ventral septal defect now has ankle pitting oedema and bi-basal crepitation in the lung fields.
5. A 13-year-old girl who has recently returned from a family holiday in India has developed night sweats, weight loss, malaise and failure to thrive.

GENERAL MEDICINE

2.6 Theme: Vitamin Deficiency

A	Vitamin A	E	Vitamin C
B	Vitamin B_1	F	Vitamin D
C	Vitamin B_6	G	Vitamin E
D	Vitamin B_{12}	H	Vitamin K

For each of the following scenarios, select the most appropriate option from the list above. You may use each option once, more than once or not at all.

1. A 65-year-old woman with a history of hypothyroidism and vitiligo has an anaemia with a mean corpuscular volume (MCV) of 102 fL. She has a positive Schilling's test.

2. A 23-year-old alcoholic with an international normalised ratio (INR) of 4.5, who is bleeding, should receive this vitamin.

3. A 95-year-old man presents to you with bleeding gums and loose teeth. You can see that his periodontal condition has worsened seriously since his last visit 12 months before. He sadly lost his wife last year and now lives on tea and biscuits.

2.7 Theme: Complications of Myocardial Infarction

A	Cardiac arrest
B	Cardiac shock
C	Dressler syndrome
D	Mitral regurgitation
E	Pericardial effusion
F	Pericarditis
G	Pulmonary embolism

For each of the following scenarios, select the most appropriate option from the list above. You may use each option once, more than once or not at all.

1. A 65-year-old woman has a massive heart attack. She has muffled heart sounds on auscultation and reduced cardiac output. On electrocardiogram (ECG) all her QRS complexes are small.

2. A 70-year-old man in the emergency department with a myocardial infarction is seen to have a change in rhythm from sinus tachycardia to an irregular broad-complex tachycardia.

3. A 32-year-old man is diagnosed in the emergency department as having an acute myocardial infarction. You look at the ECG as you are on your medical placement and the cardiologist asks what the diagnosis is. You see an ST elevation, but it is saddle-shaped.

2.8 Theme: Glasgow Coma Scale Score

A	3
B	4
C	8
D	10
E	11
F	12
G	13
H	14
I	15

For each of the following statements, choose the most appropriate Glasgow Coma Scale score from the list above. You may use each option once, more than once or not at all.

1. A patient opens his eyes to voice, localises to pain and makes incomprehensible sounds.

2. A confused nursing home resident localises to pain and opens her eyes when addressed.

3. A patient in resuscitation is found to have a 'blown and fixed pupil', is unresponsive and extends to painful stimuli.

4. A patient is shouting inappropriate words, his eyes are open and when asked to sit down, he obeys.

5. A known epileptic is assessed post-seizure and is awake and obeys commands, but his speech is slow and deliberate.

GENERAL MEDICINE

2.9 Theme: Cardiovascular Examination Findings

A Aortic regurgitation
B Aortic stenosis
C Atrial fibrillation
D Congestive cardiac failure
E Mitral regurgitation
F Mitral stenosis
G Sinus arrhythmia
H Supraventricular tachycardia
I Tricuspid regurgitation

For each of the following statements, choose the most appropriate diagnosis from the list above. You may use each option once, more than once or not at all.

1 A patient presents with cyanosis and telangiectasia. On palpation there is a parasternal heave and on auscultation a mid-diastolic murmur.

2 A known type 2 diabetic patient presents with worsening exertional dyspnoea and ankle oedema. On examination the jugular venous pressure (JVP) is raised and non-pulsatile, and there are widespread crepitations on auscultation.

3 A 50-year-old man presents following a sudden collapse at work. Examination reveals that he is in sinus rhythm and has a narrow pulse pressure.

4 A patient with a past medical history of ankylosing spondylitis is found to have a wide pulse pressure and an early diastolic murmur that is heard loudest over the left sternal edge (LSE) in expiration.

5 A 34-year-old female patient complaining of palpitations. On inspection she has a prominent goitre.

GENERAL MEDICINE

2.10 Theme: Renal Disease

A Amyloidosis
B Diabetes mellitus
C Membrano-proliferative glomerulonephritis
D Minimal change glomerulonephritis
E Multiple myeloma
F Rapidly progressing glomerulonephritis
G Renal transplant
H Sarcoidosis
I Systemic lupus erythematosus

For each of the following statements, choose the most appropriate diagnosis from the list above. You may use each option once, more than once or not at all.

1 A 56-year-old woman presents to her GP complaining of ankle swelling. A fasting blood test reveals a low-density lipoprotein (LDL) cholesterol of 4.5 mmol/l, glucose of 5.5 mmol/l, and liver function tests confirm hypoalbuminaemia.

2 A 17-year-old man presents to the emergency department complaining of excessive thirst, frequency of micturition, intermittent vomiting and abdominal pain.

3 A 41-year-old man presents with pruritus, and an abdominal examination reveals multiple suprapubic scars and a large mass in the left iliac fossa which is dull to percussion.

4 A 73-year-old patient presents with back pain. Blood tests reveal acute renal failure, hypercalcaemia and anaemia.

5 An 8-year-old child presents with nephrotic syndrome. A renal biopsy is taken, and light microscopy is unequivocal. Electron microscopy reveals fusion of podocytes.

2.11 Theme: Endocrine Disease

A   Achondroplasia
B   Acromegaly
C   Addison's disease
D   Cushing syndrome
E   Graves' disease
F   Hypothyroidism
G   Type 1 diabetes mellitus
H   Type 2 diabetes mellitus

For each of the following statements, choose the most appropriate diagnosis from the list above. You may use each option once, more than once or not at all.

1   A 76-year-old woman presents to her GP complaining of weight gain, dry brittle hair and lethargy.

2   A 19-year-old man presents to the emergency department complaining of a gradual loss of peripheral vision. On inspection of the oral cavity you notice prognathism and a large tongue.

3   A 41-year-old woman presents to the emergency department with vomiting, diarrhoea and abdominal pains. She is hypotensive and tachycardic. BM analysis reveals hypoglycaemia.

4   A 58-year-old woman with a past medical history of polymyalgia rheumatica presents with weight gain, acne and oral candidiasis.

5   A 68-year-old patient with painless jaundice and hyperglycaemia.

GENERAL MEDICINE

2.12 Theme: Examination of the Head and Neck

A	CREST syndrome
B	Dermatomyositis polymyositis
C	Fungal infection
D	Hepatitis C
E	Neurofibromatosis type 1
F	Neurofibromatosis type 2
G	Osler–Weber–Rendu syndrome
H	Rheumatoid arthritis
I	Systemic lupus erythematosus
J	Vitiligo pityriasis

For each of the following statements, choose the most appropriate diagnosis from the list above. You may use each option once, more than once or not at all.

1. A 51-year-old man presents to clinic for follow-up. On examination there are multiple café-au-lait spots and hundreds of tubular skin, neck and facial lesions.

2. A 42-year-old woman presents with violaceous rash around her eyes. She complains of blue and white hands, particularly in cold weather. On inspection she appears cachectic.

3. A 60-year-old African-American man presents with well-demarcated patches of depigmentation on his face and neck.

4. A 58-year-old woman presents with fatigue and exertional dyspnoea. Her haemoglobin is 7 g/dl and MCV 74.6. On inspection there is telangiectasia present around the mouth and under the tongue. She states that her daughter has the same problem.

5. A 46-year-old African-Caribbean woman with a butterfly rash and a recurrent history of miscarriages.

2.13 Theme: Weight Loss

A	Anorexia nervosa
B	Bulimia
C	Carcinoma of the stomach
D	Depression
E	Diabetes mellitus
F	Hypercalcaemia
G	Malabsorption
H	None of the above
I	Thyrotoxicosis
J	Tuberculosis

For each of the following scenarios, choose the most appropriate diagnosis from the list above. You may use each option once, more than once or not at all.

1. A Somali immigrant with night sweats, fever, persistent cough and weight loss.
2. A 60-year-old man with 10 kg weight loss over 4 months, epigastric discomfort, but no change in bowel habit.
3. A 35-year-old woman who opens her bowels two to three times a day, is 12 kg underweight and has angular stomatitis and oral ulceration.
4. A thin 50-year-old woman with normal appetite and atrial fibrillation.
5. A 17-year-old girl with thirst, polydipsia, polyuria and 7 kg weight loss over 3 months.

2.14 Theme: Lung Disorders

A Asthma
B Atelectasis of lung
C Bronchiectasis
D Healed fibrosed pulmonary tuberculosis
E Left ventricular failure
F Lobar pneumonia
G Pericardial effusion
H Pleural effusion
I Pneumothorax
J Pulmonary embolus

For each of the following situations, choose the most appropriate diagnosis from the list above. You may use each option once, more than once or not at all.

1 Cardiomegaly, breathlessness, bilateral basal crackles, normal chest movements and normal resonant percussion in a 75-year-old man.

2 Decreased chest movements, dullness to percussion with bronchial breathing, fever and cough productive of sputum.

3 Difficulty in breathing, over-inflated chest, resonant chest bilaterally and bilateral expiratory effort.

4 Anterior chest pain, decreased breath sounds, hyper-resonance on percussion and tactile vocal fremitus absent only on one side.

5 Decreased chest movement on one side, dullness to percussion, absent breath sounds and absent tactile vocal fremitus.

2.15 Theme: Back Pain

A Ankylosing spondylitis
B Bony metastases
C Cauda equina syndrome
D L 3/4 disc with L4 signs
E L 4/5 disc with S1 signs
F Paget's disease
G Spinal cord compression
H Tuberculosis of the spine
I Vertebral crush fracture

For each of the following scenarios, choose the most appropriate diagnosis from the list above. You may use each option once, more than once or not at all.

1 A 65-year-old woman with long-standing back pain. She presents with an exacerbation of the pain, urinary retention, saddle anaesthesia and absent ankle jerks.

2 A 60-year-old woman, who has been treated with steroids for 15 years, presents with sudden-onset, severe back pain.

3 A 75-year-old man with a 3-month history of 10 kg weight loss and back pain which is worse at night.

4 A 20-year-old with lower back pain but an extremely high erythrocyte sedimentation rate (ESR).

5 A 25-year-old banker with acute-onset, severe low back pain. He has left-sided sciatica and an absent left ankle jerk.

2.16 Theme: Abdominal Masses

A   Aortic aneurysm
B   Carcinoma of the caecum
C   Carcinoma of the stomach
D   Gall bladder disease
E   Hepatomegaly
F   Inguinal hernia
G   Pancreatic pseudocyst
H   Polycystic kidneys
I   Splenomegaly

For each of the following scenarios, choose the most appropriate diagnosis from the list above. You may use each option once, more than once or not at all.

1   A 56-year-old man with jaundice, spider naevi and a right upper quadrant mass.
2   A 69-year-old woman with an upper left quadrant pass and lymphadenopathy.
3   A 45-year-old woman with bilateral loin masses. She has both personal and family history of loin pain and hypertension.
4   A 75-year-old man with sudden severe abdominal pain and an expansile, pulsatile central abdominal mass.
5   A 74-year-old woman with iron deficiency and a right iliac fossa mass.

2.17 Theme: Diabetic Complications

A   Arteriopathy
B   Arthropathy
C   Autonomic neuropathy
D   Charcot arthropathy
E   Haemoglobinopathy
F   Ischaemic heart disease
G   Nephropathy
H   Peripheral neuropathy
I   Retinopathy
J   Uropathy

For each of the following scenarios, choose the most appropriate diabetic complication from the list above. You may use each option once, more than once or not at all.

1   A 60-year-old man with three cold and black toes.
2   An 80-year-old with raised urea and creatinine.
3   A 70-year-old man with gallop rhythm and intermittent nocturnal breathlessness.
4   A 68-year-old man with no sensation to pinprick up to the knee.
5   A 75-year-old man with postural hypertension.

2.18 Theme: Liver

- **A** Alcoholic liver disease
- **B** Congestive cardiac failure
- **C** Epstein–Barr virus infection
- **D** Glycogen storage disease
- **E** Haemochromatosis
- **F** Hepatitis B
- **G** Liver abscess
- **H** Metastatic liver disease
- **I** Primary liver cell cancer

For each of the following scenarios, choose the most appropriate diagnosis from the list above. You may use each option once, more than once or not at all.

1. A 46-year-old publican with spider naevi, bruising, confusion and jaundice.
2. A 27-year-old intravenous drug user with fever and abdominal pain.
3. A 50-year-old woman with pigmented skin, type 1 diabetes mellitus and raised transaminases.
4. A 50-year-old woman with jaundice 3 years after chemotherapy for breast cancer.
5. A 75-year-old man with shortness of breath, raised jugular venous pressure (JVP) and swollen legs.

2.19 Theme: Lymphadenopathy

A Carcinoma of the lung
B Chronic lymphocytic leukaemia
C Epstein–Barr virus infection
D Hodgkin's lymphoma
E Human immunodeficiency virus (HIV) infection
F Rheumatoid arthritis
G Sarcoidosis
H Systemic lupus erythematosus (SLE)
I Toxoplasmosis
J Tuberculous lymphadenitis

For each of the following scenarios, choose the most appropriate diagnosis from the list above. You may use each option once, more than once or not at all.

1 An 18-year-old female with a 3-week history of sore throat, fever, malaise and enlarged lymph nodes.

2 A 45-year-old smoker with 15 kg weight loss and finger clubbing.

3 A 25-year-old Asian man with fever, night sweats and a single cervical lymph node.

4 A 65-year-old man with a large spleen and markedly raised white cell count.

5 A 30-year-old woman with bilateral facial rash, fever and joint pain.

2.20 Theme: Abdominal Distension

A	Ascites
B	Carcinoma of the colon
C	Crohn disease
D	Distended bladder
E	Flatus
F	Ileus
G	Large bowel obstruction
H	Liver metastases
I	Ovarian tumour
J	Peritonitis
K	Pregnancy
L	Small bowel obstruction

For each of the following situations, choose the most appropriate cause for abdominal distension from the list above. You may use each option once, more than once or not at all.

1. A distended abdomen with dullness to percussion. There is also dullness in the flanks and in the suprapubic region. The dullness shifts from side to side when you roll the patient.

2. A distended abdomen with a 2-day history of vomiting, central abdominal pain, increased bowel sounds and no faeces or flatus.

3. A distended abdomen in a patient who lies still with rebound tenderness, guarding and no bowel sounds.

4. A distended midline mass arising from the pelvis in a postmenopausal woman with no urinary symptoms.

5. A distended tympanic abdomen, 4 days after abdominal surgery with no bowel sounds and no flatus.

2.21 Theme: Loss of Consciousness

A Complete heart block
B Epileptic seizure
C Hyperventilation
D Hypoglycaemia
E Hysterical fugue state
F Infarction of cerebral hemisphere
G Subarachnoid haemorrhage
H Transient ischaemic attack
I Vasovagal faint
J Vertebrobasilar ischaemia

For each of the following scenarios, choose the most appropriate diagnosis from the list above. You may use each option once, more than once or not at all.

1. A 45-year-old man who has had three episodes where he has lost consciousness and fallen to the ground. He has no recollection of the incident, but bit his tongue and was incontinent to urine.

2. A 25-year-old woman with breathing difficulties, light-headedness and carpopedal spasm.

3. A 79-year-old man who lost the ability to speak for 2 hours, but is now neurologically normal.

4. A 79-year-old woman who has dizzy spells when looking up to hang out washing.

5. A 37-year-old man with sudden-onset, severe headache in the occiput region collapses.

GENERAL MEDICINE

2.22 Theme: Chest Pain

A   Angina
B   Aortic aneurysm
C   Myocardial infarction
D   Oesophagitis
E   Pericarditis
F   Pneumonia
G   Pulmonary embolism
H   Unstable angina
I   Zoster

For each of the following scenarios, choose the most appropriate diagnosis from the list above. You may use each option once, more than once or not at all.

1 A 60-year-old with acute severe chest pain radiating through to the back with a wide mediastinum on chest X-ray.

2 A 75-year-old smoker with central chest pain radiating to the jaw when he walks to the shops. This pain resolves at rest.

3 A 40-year-old woman with right-sided chest pain, worse on breathing in. There is associated coughing and haemoptysis.

4 A 53-year-old man with sudden-onset chest pain, radiating to the left arm, associated with sweating and nausea. This pain has been present for 2 hours.

5 A 76-year-old obese man with episodes of low retrosternal burning pain, and difficulty swallowing.

2.23 Theme: Eye Disease

A   III nerve palsy
B   VI nerve palsy
C   Brainstem death
D   Expanding pituitary tumour
E   Horner syndrome
F   Large right-sided cerebral hemisphere tumour
G   Left-sided cerebral hemisphere infarction
H   Opiate overdose
I   Thyroid eye disease

For each of the following situations, choose the most appropriate diagnosis from the list above. You may use each option once, more than once or not at all.

1 Bilateral pinpoint pupils in a comatose young patient.

2 Right-sided homonymous hemianopia.

3 Eye deviated downwards and outwards with ptosis and large pupil.

4 Bronchial carcinoma with ptosis and small pupil.

5 Fixed and dilated pupils after resuscitation.

2.24 Theme: Abdominal Pain

A Aortic aneurysm pain
B Appendicitis
C Biliary colic
D Duodenal ulcer
E Gastro-oesophageal reflux disease
F Pancreatitis
G Renal colic
H Small-bowel colic
I Uterine pain

For each of the following situations, choose the most likely cause for the abdominal pain from the list above. You may use each option once, more than once or not at all.

1 Left loin and left upper quadrant pain radiating to the groin.
2 Epigastric and low retrosternal pain associated with food regurgitation.
3 Epigastric and right upper quadrant pain radiating to the infrascapular region.
4 Gripping abdominal pain (central) that comes and goes over short periods of time.
5 Epigastric pain that is worse when hungry, awakens the patient at night and is relieved by milk.

2.25 Theme: Collapse

A   Alcohol intoxication
B   Complete heart block
C   Epilepsy
D   Gram-negative sepsis
E   Left ventricular failure
F   Mechanical fall
G   Meningococcal sepsis
H   Pulmonary embolism
I   Supraventricular tachycardia
J   Vasovagal faint

For each of the following scenarios, choose the most appropriate diagnosis from the list above. You may use each option once, more than once or not at all.

1   80-year-old man with shortness of breath and crackles in both lung fields collapses.

2   An 18-year-old man acutely and severely ill. He has low blood pressure, neck stiffness and purpura.

3   A 36-year-old woman collapses in a postnatal ward 4 days after a caesarean section. She has raised neck veins, hypoxia and haemoptysis.

4   A 75-year-old woman with recurrent urinary tract infections presents severely ill with an unrecordable blood pressure. She has blood, protein and nitrites in her urine.

5   An 18-year-old brought in via ambulance after collapsing on an underground train in London. On examination she is alert and well and her pulse and blood pressure is normal.

2.26 Theme: Hand Signs

A	Capillary dilatation	F	Leuconychia
B	Clubbing	G	Osler nodes
C	Dupuytren contracture	H	Pitted finger nails
D	Heberden nodes	I	Raynaud phenomenon
E	Koilonychia	J	Trigger finger

For each of the following scenarios, choose the most appropriate hand sign from the list above. You may use each option once, more than once or not at all.

1. A 25-year-old man with infective endocarditis.
2. A 73-year-old with squamous cell carcinoma of the bronchus.
3. A 25-year-old with hypoalbuminaemia from nephritic syndrome.
4. A 58-year-old with generalised osteoarthritis.
5. A 47-year-old with psoriasis.

2.27 Theme: General Conditions

A	Addison's disease
B	Anaemia
C	Anxiety
D	Depression
E	Fibromyalgia
F	Hypothyroidism
G	Infective arthritis
H	Thyrotoxicosis
I	Tuberculosis
J	Wegener granulomatosis

For each of the following scenarios, choose the most appropriate diagnosis from the list above. You may use each option once, more than once or not at all.

1. A 27-year-old woman with weight loss, shortness of breath, nose bleeds, haemoptysis and skin rash.
2. A 25-year-old woman, agitated with tachycardia and exophthalmos.
3. A 65-year-old woman with paucity of speech, early morning waking and flat affect.
4. A 50-year-old man taking warfarin complains of tiredness. He has haematuria and exertional breathlessness, and is apyrexic.
5. A 40-year-old with poor sleep pattern, aches, pains and trigger points.

2.28 Theme: Diarrhoea and Vomiting

A	Amoebic dysentery
B	Cholera
C	Coeliac disease
D	Hepatitis A
E	Irritable bowel syndrome
F	Lactose intolerance
G	Norwalk virus infection
H	Rotavirus infection
I	*Salmonella* infection
F	Ulcerative colitis

For each of the following scenarios, choose the most appropriate diagnosis from the list above. You may use each option once, more than once or not at all.

1 A 25-year-old engineer working in Sierra Leone has abdominal pain, bloody diarrhoea and an enlarged liver.

2 A 50-year-old couple on a Caribbean cruise, with sudden-onset diarrhoea and vomiting. Another 50 people on the boat have similar symptoms.

3 A volunteer returns from a Rwanda refugee camp with watery diarrhoea, associated flakes and mucus, and dehydration.

4 An 8-month-old baby with mild dehydration, a 1-day history of malaise, irritability and diarrhoea. Several other children attending the same crèche have similar symptoms.

5 A 2-year-old with diarrhoea and vomiting after eating soft boiled eggs on a farm holiday.

GENERAL MEDICINE

2.29 Theme: Respiratory Diagnosis

A   Acute coronary syndrome
B   Asthma
C   Aspiration pneumonia
D   Chronic obstructive pulmonary disease
E   Fibrosing alveolitis
F   Hyperventilation
G   Pneumonia
H   Pulmonary embolus
I   Pulmonary oedema
J   Respiratory muscle weakness

For each of the following scenarios, choose the most appropriate diagnosis from the list above. You may use each option once, more than once or not at all.

1. A 72-year-old with motor neurone disease and progressive breathlessness over 12 months.
2. A 25-year-old with short episodes of breathlessness, principally at rest or when speaking in public.
3. A 76-year-old woman with a 12-month history of end-inspiratory bilateral crackles with normal left ventricular function.
4. A 35-year-old with breathlessness and wheezing.
5. A 50-year-old with a 24-hour history of gradually worsening pleuritic chest pain and a temperature of 40°C.

2.30 Theme: Infections

A *Bordetella pertussis*
B *Candida albicans*
C Cytomegalovirus
D Herpes simplex virus
E *Mycobacterium tuberculosis*
F *Pneumocystis carinii*
G Respiratory syncytial virus
H *Streptococcus pneumoniae*
I *Treponema pallidum*
J Varicella zoster

For each of the following scenarios, choose the most appropriate causative organism from the list above. You may use each option once, more than once or not at all.

1 A bone marrow recipient, 2 months after transplant, presents with fever, leucopenia, hypoxia and interstitial infiltrations in the lungs which can be seen on a chest X-ray. He has increased respiratory rate and rib retraction.

2 A 6-month-old baby with wheeze, cyanosis, rapid breathing and rib retraction.

3 A 45-year-old smoker with chronic obstructive pulmonary disease, with pleuritic chest pain, rusty sputum, shortness of breath and rapid respiratory rate.

4 A Bangladeshi immigrant with productive cough, weight loss, low grade fever and malaise.

5 A 40-year-old drug misuser with rapid breathing and bilateral lung infiltrates.

GENERAL MEDICINE

2.31 Theme: Endocrine Conditions

A	Acromegaly	F	Hypogonadism
B	Conn disease	G	Hypothyroidism
C	Cushing disease	H	Prolactinoma
D	Diabetes insipidus	I	TSH-oma
E	Growth hormone deficiency	J	Type 1 diabetes

For each of the following scenarios, choose the most appropriate diagnosis from the list above. You may use each option once, more than once or not at all.

1. A 40-year-old woman who is hypertensive, obese, with striae and has difficulty getting up from a chair.
2. A patient with bipolar affective disorder, polyuria and a low urine osmolality.
3. A large woman with hyperhidrosis, headaches and carpal tunnel syndrome. Her condition was diagnosed following an oral glucose tolerance test.
4. A 27-year-old woman with galactorrhoea.
5. A 59-year-old woman with a history of weight gain, dry hair and constipation.

2.32 Theme: Severe Infections

A	Brain abscess	F	Osteomyelitis
B	Cystitis	G	Peritonitis
C	Infective endocarditis	H	Post-operative pneumonia
D	Influenza	I	Post-operative wound infection
E	Meningococcal septicaemia	J	Pyelonephritis

For each of the following scenarios, choose the most appropriate infective condition from the list above. You may use each option once, more than once or not at all.

1. A 20-year-old man who is not arousable has a purpuric rash on his legs.
2. A 5-year-old girl with fever and pain in her right thigh for the past 2 days. She will not weight-bear on her right leg.
3. A 20-year-old woman with acute-onset fever, rigors and loin pain.
4. A 60-year-old man with a changing arrhthymia and a 2-month history of fever and malaise.
5. A 55-year-old man with fever and worsening abdominal pain following laparoscopic abdominal surgery 6 hours previously.

2.33 Theme: Lower-limb Problems

A   Cellulitis
B   Congestive cardiac failure
C   Deep vein thrombosis
D   Dependent oedema
E   Lymphoedema
F   Necrotising fasciitis
G   Nephritic syndrome
H   Ruptured Baker cyst
I   Superficial thrombophlebitis

For each of the following scenarios, choose the most appropriate diagnosis from the list above. You may use each option once, more than once or not at all.

1   A 28-year-old pregnant woman with left leg pain and swelling.

2   A 65-year-old fit and well woman with swelling of both ankles which is worse at the end of the day, but is not present on rising in the morning.

3   A 75-year-old man with ischaemic heart disease with bilateral leg swelling up to the knees, and associated shortness of breath.

4   A 30-year-old woman with worsening swelling of both legs over 2 weeks, raised cholesterol and low protein level.

5   A 45-year-old diabetic man with a swollen painful leg 2 days after an insect bite. The overlying skin is red and painful to touch.

2.34 Theme: Pre-operative Investigations

A   Abdominal ultrasound
B   Cervical spine X-ray
C   Chest X-ray
D   Coagulation screen
E   Echocardiogram
F   Electrocardiogram (ECG)
G   Endoscopic retrograde cholangiopancreatography (ERCP)
H   Exercise stress test
I   Full blood count
J   Spirometry

For each of the following scenarios, choose the most appropriate investigation from the list above. You may use each option once, more than once or not at all.

1. A 46-year-old woman undergoing a minor gynaecological procedure for heavy periods.

2. A 58-year-old man undergoing an arthroscopy on his right knee. He is currently taking warfarin for deep vein thrombosis which occurred 3 months ago.

3. A 55-year-old man who smokes, has a productive cough and has finger clubbing. Surgery on his varicose veins is planned.

4. A 75-year-old woman with rheumatoid arthritis requiring intubation and an anaesthetic for hip replacement.

5. A patient awaiting gall bladder removal develops jaundice, raised bilirubin and raised alkaline phosphatase.

GENERAL MEDICINE

2.35 Theme: Infections of the Lung

A	*Aspergillus fumigatus*	F	*Mycobacterium tuberculosis*
B	Cytomegalovirus	G	*Mycoplasma pneumoniae*
C	Influenza	H	*Pneumocystis carinii*
D	*Legionella pneumophila*	I	*Pseudomonas aeruginosa*
E	Measles	J	*Staphylococcus aureus*

For each of the following scenarios, choose the most appropriate option from the list above. You may use each option once, more than once or not at all.

1 A 59-year-old homeless man with weight loss, sweats and fever.

2 A 71-year-old man with pneumonia who has been at a 3-day conference in a poorly kept hotel.

3 A 28-year-old HIV-infected man with pneumonia.

4 A 28-year-old man on co-trimoxazole prophylaxis after renal transplantation develops pneumonia.

5 A 17-year-old boy with cystic fibrosis develops pneumonia with cavitation.

2.36 Theme: Tests

A	Alkaline phosphatase	F	Plasma glucose
B	Amylase	G	Protein electrophoresis
C	Bilirubin	H	Synacthen test
D	Calcium	I	Thyroxine (T4)
E	Iron studies	J	Vitamin D

For each of the following scenarios, choose the most appropriate diagnostic test from the list above. You may use each option once, more than once or not at all.

1 A 50-year-old obese man with angina.

2 A 44-year-old woman with a 6-year history of fatigue, hand tremor and palpitations. Her ECG shows sinus tachycardia and atrial fibrillation.

3 A 76-year-old woman with a long history of worsening hip and thigh pain. A pelvic X-ray shows marked sclerosis and lucency in the right hemi-pelvis.

4 An 80-year-old man with bone pain, abdominal discomfort, kidney stones and occasional psychosis.

5 A 50-year-old alcoholic with severe central abdominal pain. He has been hospitalised for this problem before.

2.1 Eating Disorders

1　C　Bulimia

2　H　Reflux oesophagitis

3　G　Plummer–Vinson syndrome

4　F　Pharyngeal pouch

5　B　Anorexia

Bulimics are frequently of normal weight but cause voluntary vomiting in order to control their weight. The acid attack on the teeth causes palatal tooth wear on the incisor teeth and frequently on the occlusal surfaces of the molars.

Anorexics are usually very underweight but do not recognise that they need to put weight on. Anorexics usually do not eat sufficient calories and do not usually have voluntary regurgitation.

Reflux oesophagitis is commonly associated with excessive salivation.

Plummer–Vinson syndrome, also known as Patterson–Brown–Kelly syndrome, is an iron deficiency anaemia that causes spoon-shaped finger nails (koilonychia). Glossitis and angular stomatitis are also common in these patients.

Pharyngeal pouch causes swelling and difficulty in swallowing.

GENERAL MEDICINE

2.2 HIV/AIDS

1 D Epstein–Barr virus (EBV)

2 E Human herpesvirus 8

3 A *Candida albicans*

4 C Cytomegalovirus (CMV)

5 F *Streptococcus*

Intracerebral Hodgkin's lymphoma is associated with Epstein–Barr virus in HIV patients, as is Kaposi's sarcoma with human herpesvirus 8.

Odynophagia (painful swallowing) may indicate a *Candida* infection in the immunocompromised. Cytomegalovirus (CMV) can cause retinitis, and streptococcal pneumonia is the most frequent type in HIV patients.

2.3 UK Malignancy Death Rate

1 B 10 000

2 C 15 000

3 G 35 000

4 B 10 000

5 A 5000

6 B 10 000

Note that breast, prostate and lymphoma have a similar death rate per annum.

In the UK the Office for National Statistics publishes the incidence for malignancies within the four UK countries. The incidence does vary across the UK, with Wales having a 6% and Scotland a 15% higher incidence of malignancy than the whole of the UK. The incidence does vary slightly year to year.

GENERAL MEDICINE

2.4 Personality Disorders

1	F	Narcissism
2	H	Schizoid
3	C	Borderline
4	D	Dependent
5	G	Obsessive-compulsive

Affective disorder is characterised by dramatic changes or extremes of mood, including mania or depression.

Anxious personality disorder is a condition characterised by extreme shyness, feelings of inadequacy, and sensitivity to rejection.

Histrionic personality disorder is characterised by a long-standing pattern of attention-seeking behaviour and extreme emotionality.

2.5 Shortness of Breath in Children

1	B	Croup
2	D	Inhaled foreign body
3	G	Whooping cough
4	C	Heart failure
5	F	Tuberculosis

Acute asthma may cause wheezing and shortness of breath, but the noise is different from whooping cough (pertussis). Symptoms with asthma are usually worse at night or early morning. Croup tends to be worse at night. Children with heart failure usually have difficulty breathing, low blood pressure and excessive sweating. Ankle oedema with pitting is also a sign of heart failure. Ankle swelling which is non-pitting may occur in conditions such as hypothyroidism, when the tissues are thickened but not due to fluid retention. Inhaled foreign bodies may result in persistent coughs in children, and inhalation should be suspected if it has occurred after a recent choking event. The majority of children who inhale foreign bodies are usually between 1 and 3 years old. Due to the right bronchus being straighter (ie more in line with the trachea), inhaled foreign bodies are more likely to end in the right side, and hence they are unilateral. Childhood pneumonias follow infections and are usually associated with a cough and high temperature. Tuberculosis is still prevalent in many parts of the developing world and should be suspected in children with persistent coughs who have recent been in such countries.

2.6 Vitamin Deficiency

1 D Vitamin B_{12}

She has pernicious anaemia, which is the most commonest cause of B_{12} deficiency. It is common in the elderly and more so females. There is an association with other autoimmune disease such as vitiligo, thyroid disease and Addison's disease. Usually a megaloblastic anaemia is found and the Schilling test is diagnostic.

2 H Vitamin K

Vitamin K is a cofactor essential for the blood-clotting factors, other proteins in coagulation and also for proteins for the formation of bone.

3 E Vitamin C

Presentation of this disease can be very non-specific; elderly who are malnourished can often succumb to vitamin C deficiency. The symptoms can be very variable, commonly though spongy or swollen bleeding gums with loose teeth are a sign picked up if the individual is a regular dental attender often with recurrent infections and haemorrhage.

GENERAL MEDICINE

2.7 Complications of Myocardial Infarction

1 E Pericardial effusion

The fluid reduces the heart's ability to beat, as represented on the ECG.

2 A Cardiac arrest

This patient has ventricular fibrillation.

3 F Pericarditis

This is the classic ECG change for pericarditis.

2.8 Glasgow Coma Scale Score

1 D Score 10

2 F Score 12

3 B Score 4

4 G Score 13

5 H Score 14

The Glasgow Coma Scale score is measured from 3 up to a complete score of 15.

- Eye opening: none: 1, to pain: 2, to speech: 3, spontaneously: 4.
- Verbal: none: 1, incomprehensible sounds: 2, inappropriate words: 3, confused: 4, orientated: 5
- Motor: none: 1, extension to pain: 2, abnormal flexion to pain: 3, withdraws from pain: 4, localises to pain: 5, obeys commands: 6

2.9 Cardiovascular Examination Findings

1 F Mitral stenosis

Mitral stenosis (MS) is most often caused by rheumatic heart disease. Many patients with MS will be in atrial fibrillation and facially exhibit a malar flush (cyanosis and telangiectasia). Mitral valve repair is the treatment of choice.

2 D Congestive cardiac failure

This patient presents with symptoms of both right-sided heart failure (ankle oedema) and left-sided heart failure (pulmonary oedema). Ischaemic heart disease is a common cause and this patient has a significant risk factor as they have diabetes mellitus type 2.

3 B Aortic stenosis

Patients with AS can present complaining of shortness of breath/chest pain or syncope. A low systolic with a narrow pulse pressure and an ejection systolic murmur that radiates to the carotids are common findings. Bicuspid valves and rheumatic heart disease are causes.

4 A Aortic regurgitation

In this case ankylosing spondylitis is the cause of AR, and other causes include rheumatoid arthritis, rheumatic fever and infective endocarditis. Common examination findings include a collapsing pulse, a wide pulse pressure and an early diastolic murmur.

5 C Atrial fibrillation

Irregular pulse. Associated with MS, drugs, alcohol and in this case hyperthyroidism/thyrotoxicosis.

2.10 Renal Disease

1 I Systemic lupus erythematosus (SLE)

This woman presents with nephrotic syndrome; causes include autoimmune disorders/diabetes/malignancy and drugs. In this case SLE is the cause in light of the normal fasting glucose result, excluding diabetes.

2 B Diabetes mellitus

This is a common first presentation of diabetic ketoacidosis, ie type 1 diabetes mellitus. Arterial blood gas sampling will reveal metabolic acidosis and a high blood sugar.

3 G Renal transplant

This is a common site for a renal transplant.

4 E Multiple myeloma

This is consistent with the haematological malignancy – multiple myeloma. Hypercalcaemia is caused by activation of osteoclasts which cause the lytic lesions on plain radiograph. Acute renal failure may be secondary to hypercalcaemia or due to aggregation of overproduced monoclonal light chains congregating in the glomeruli. Bence Jones proteins may be found on urinalysis.

5 D Minimal change glomerulonephritis

Minimal change glomerulonephritis is the commonest cause of nephrotic syndrome in children and usually responds to steroids.

2.11   Endocrine Disease

1   F   Hypothyroidism

These are typical complaints of patients with hypothyroidism.

2   B   Acromegaly

Acromegaly is most commonly caused by a growth hormone-secreting pituitary adenoma that is active after puberty when the growth plates of the long bones have already fused. Other features include large hands, prominent brow and jaw, macroglossia and a broad nose. A pituitary adenoma may also cause bitemporal hemianopia secondary to compression of the optic nerve decussation.

3   C   Addison's disease

This presentation is consistent with an addisonian crisis, ie severe failure of the adrenals to produce steroid hormones, particularly cortisol. A crisis may be precipitated by intercurrent infection.

4   D   Cushing syndrome

Patients with polymyalgia rheumatica may be commenced on steroids if their symptoms fail to respond to non-steroidal anti-inflammatory drugs (NSAIDs). Long-term steroid therapy can give rise to cushingoid features such as acne, hirsutism, a buffalo hump, striae. Patients are typically at increased risk of infection and are also hyperglycaemic.

5   G   Type 1 diabetes mellitus

Painless jaundice and late-onset diabetes in the elderly may be suggestive of pancreatic cancer.

2.12 Examination of the Head and Neck

1 E Neurofibromatosis (NF) type 1

This is inherited in an autosomal dominant manner. Clinically there is also axillary freckling and there may be visual/auditory problems associated with neurofibromas on the cranial nerves. Type 2 NF presents without skin lesions.

2 B Dermatomyositis polymyositis

This is a disease of unknown aetiology, although it is often found in mixed connective tissue disease. The heliotrope rash, muscular weakness and pain are common complaints along with Raynaud's phenomenon. There is a strong link with underlying malignancy and this should be investigated promptly. Diagnosis of dermatomyositis polymyositis is confirmed with muscle biopsy.

3 J Vitiligo pityriasis

This is typical of vitiligo. Vitiligo is associated with diabetes, Addison's disease, alopecia and thyroid disease.

4 G Osler-Weber-Rendu syndrome

This is also known as hereditary haemorrhagic telangiectasia (autosomal dominant). Patients often present with recurrent epistaxis and anaemia (occurs with gastrointestinal arteriovenous malformations and multiple telangiectasias).

5 I Systemic lupus erythematosus (SLE)

SLE is a chronic inflammatory disease that affects the blood vessels and connective tissues of the skin and various parts of the body. There is also a simple form called 'discoid lupus' which just affects the skin.

GENERAL MEDICINE

2.13 Weight Loss

1	J	Tuberculosis
2	C	Carcinoma of the stomach
3	G	Malabsorption
4	I	Thyrotoxicosis
5	E	Diabetes mellitus

Night sweats, fever, persistent cough and weight loss is the classic picture of tuberculosis. Tuberculosis is diagnosed by a combination of Mantoux test, sputum culture and chest X-ray. It is a communicable disease and is treated with rifampicin, isoniazid, pyrazinamide and ethambutol. In Q 2 the age, epigastric discomfort and weight loss of 10 kg points to stomach cancer. The 35-year-old woman is underweight, but the question does not state that she has lost weight. She has symptoms of iron deficiency, and this points to malabsorption. Atrial fibrillation is a common symptom of thyrotoxicosis, and must be treated with warfarin and digoxin. Thirst, polyuria and weight loss in a young person is a typical presentation of diabetes.

2.14 Lung Disorders

1	E	Left ventricular failure
2	F	Lobar pneumonia
3	A	Asthma
4	I	Pneumothorax
5	H	Pleural effusion

It is important to look for the key words in this EMQ. The mention of cardiomegaly and breathlessness is indicative of cardiac failure, therefore left ventricular failure. The mention of fever and productive sputum is indicative of infection, and therefore pneumonia. The difficulty in breathing, over-inflated chest and bilateral expiratory effort is classic of asthma. Hyper-resonance is a key word for pneumothorax.

2.15 Back Pain

ANSWERS

1	C	Cauda equina syndrome
2	I	Vertebral crush fracture
3	B	Bony metastases
4	A	Ankylosing spondylitis
5	E	L 4/5 disc with S1 signs

The hint for cauda equina syndrome is the mention of saddle anaesthesia. The link is that 'equina' means 'horse' in Latin, and this is the link with saddle. The 60-year-old woman on long-term steroid treatment is demonstrating the long-term effects of steroids, one of which is osteoporosis. People with osteoporosis are at risk of vertebral crush fracture from their own weight. The raised ESR and back pain in a young man is highly indicative of ankylosing spondylitis. A history of acute weight loss in older people is frequently indicative of cancer. The young banker who has unilateral pain and neurological symptoms in an atraumatic scenario is likely to have a prolapsed disc. The lack of an ankle jerk is an S1 sign.

2.16 Abdominal Masses

1	E	Hepatomegaly
2	I	Splenomegaly
3	H	Polycystic kidneys
4	A	Aortic aneurysm
5	B	Carcinoma of the caecum

The key to this question is having knowledge of where organs are in the abdomen. Jaundice and a right upper quadrant mass is indicative of liver disease. In the left upper quadrant the spleen is present. Bilateral loin pain is usually from the kidneys. Polycystic kidneys have a hereditary component and cause hypertension. When pulsatile is mentioned, it is associated with blood vessels. A central pulsatile mass with pain is indicative of a dissecting aortic aneurysm. Malabsorption of iron and a mass in the right iliac fossa is the classic history of cancer of the caecum.

2.17 Diabetic Complications

1	A	Arteriopathy
2	G	Nephropathy
3	F	Ischaemic heart disease
4	H	Peripheral neuropathy
5	C	Autonomic neuropathy

The black toes are indicative of gangrene, and therefore poor blood supply. Raised urea and creatinine are associated with renal failure. The gallop rhythm and nocturnal breathlessness are signs of heart failure. The lack of pinprick sensation is related to peripheral neuropathy, whereas the inability to control blood pressure on standing is indicative of an autonomic problem.

2.18 Liver

1 A Alcoholic liver disease

2 F Hepatitis B

3 E Haemochromatosis

4 H Metastatic liver disease

5 B Congestive cardiac failure

The signs of alcoholic liver disease are jaundice, spider naevi, bruising and confusion. The bruising occurs because liver cirrhosis prevents formation of clotting factors; the confusion is because of the lack of thiamine absorption, leading to Wernicke encephalopathy and Korsakoff syndrome. The intravenous drug user is a give-away for hepatitis B because of sharing of needles. Haemochromatosis is an autosomal recessive condition where iron absorption is not regulated and there is excessive absorption of iron. This is deposited in various organs, including the heart, liver, pancreas and skin. This leads to the classic bronze (skin) diabetes (deposition of iron in the pancreas). Breast cancer metastasises to the liver and also to bone. The shortness of breath, swollen legs and raised JVP are signs of cardiac failure.

2.19 Lymphadenopathy

1 C Epstein–Barr virus infection

2 A Carcinoma of the lung

3 J Tuberculous lymphadenitis

4 B Chronic lymphocytic leukaemia

5 H SLE

Epstein–Barr virus infection is known as the 'kissing disease' and this is the most likely diagnosis in Q 1. The weight loss and clubbing indicates cancer. The night sweats, fever and lymphadenopathy are classic of tuberculosis. Splenomegaly and raised white cell count in an elderly person should make the clinician think of chronic lymphocytic leukaemia. A bilateral or butterfly facial rash makes SLE the likely diagnosis.

GENERAL MEDICINE

2.20 Abdominal Distension

| 1 | A | Ascites |

| 2 | L | Small bowel obstruction |

| 3 | J | Peritonitis |

| 4 | I | Ovarian tumour |

| 5 | F | Ileus |

There are five main causes of a distended abdomen: fat, fluid, fetus, faeces and flatus. Statement A is a textbook definition of ascites. If a patient has no bowel sounds, faeces or flatus, it means that there is either a blockage or there is no bowel peristalsis (ileus). Ileus is common after surgery. Ovarian tumours often cause fluid retention and a distended abdomen.

2.21 Loss of Consciousness

| 1 | B | Epileptic seizure |

| 2 | C | Hyperventilation |

| 3 | H | Transient ischaemic attack |

| 4 | J | Vertebrobasilar ischaemia |

| 5 | G | Subarachnoid haemorrhage |

A young woman with breathlessness and carpopedal spasm is indicative of hyperventilation. When somebody looks upwards the vertebrobasilar arteries are compressed, and if they are insufficient, it leads to dizziness. A transient ischaemic attack is described as the production of a neurological deficit which resolves within 24 hours. A patient who has a severe headache and collapses is most likely to have a subarachnoid haemorrhage.

2.22 Chest Pain

1 B Aortic aneurysm

2 A Angina

3 G Pulmonary embolism

4 C Myocardial infarction

5 D Oesophagitis

Angina if it is unstable occurs at rest. If it is of effort it resolves by resting. Myocardial infarction is suspected if pain is present for greater than 20 minutes, and it is associated with sweating and nausea. If there is fever, pneumonia is suspected, however, in Q 3 there is pain and haemoptysis, which indicates pulmonary embolism. Also be aware that not all chest pain is cardiac-related. It can be muscular, infective (zoster) and often can be related to gastric conditions.

2.23 Eye Disease

1 H Opiate overdose

2 G Left-sided cerebral hemisphere infarction

3 A III nerve palsy

4 E Horner syndrome

5 C Brainstem death

A young person with pinpoint pupils usually means an opiate overdose. If there is a right-sided homonymous hemianopia, it is likely that there is a left cerebral hemisphere lesion or bleed. Horner syndrome is caused by interruption of the sympathetic nerve supply to the face. The fixed and dilated pupils mean brainstem death.

GENERAL MEDICINE

2.24 Abdominal Pain

1 G Renal colic

2 E Gastro-oesophageal reflux disease

3 C Biliary colic

4 H Small-bowel colic

5 D Duodenal ulcer

Duodenal ulcers are worse at meal times and are relieved by milk.

2.25 Collapse

1 E Left ventricular failure

2 G Meningococcal sepsis

3 H Pulmonary embolism

4 D Gram-negative sepsis

5 J Vasovagal faint

The classic signs of meningism are neck stiffness, purpura, and fever. Pulmonary embolism is a surgical complication. Gram-negative sepsis is a very serious condition associated with urinary tract infections, as these are caused by Gram-negative organisms.

2.26 Hand Signs

1 G Osler nodes

2 B Clubbing

3 F Leuconychia

4 D Heberden nodes

5 H Pitted finger nails

Rheumatic fever is associated with petechiae, Osler nodes and Janeway lesions. A bronchial carcinoma is associated with clubbing and the patient may show the Horner sign. Heberden nodes are found on the fingers of patients with osteoarthritis.

2.27 General Conditions

1 J Wegener granulomatosis

2 H Thyrotoxicosis

3 D Depression

4 B Anaemia

5 E Fibromyalgia

Wegener granulomatosis is a potentially fatal granulomatous vasculitis, which affects many systems. If a patient is taking warfarin, they may not be taking it correctly and may have a high international normalised ratio (INR), leading to bleeding and therefore anaemia. Fibromyalgia is classically described as a condition with painful trigger points, sore joints and difficulty sleeping.

GENERAL MEDICINE   87

2.28 Diarrhoea and Vomiting

1   A   Amoebic dysentery

2   G   Norwalk virus infection

3   B   Cholera

4   H   Rotavirus infection

5   I   *Salmonella* infection

Watery diarrhoea occurs in cholera, and bloody diarrhoea occurs in amoebic dysentery. Norwalk virus infection is common on cruise ships. Rotavirus is common in young children, and *Salmonella* infection is associated with eggs.

2.29 Respiratory Diagnosis

1   J   Respiratory muscle weakness

2   F   Hyperventilation

3   E   Fibrosing alveolitis

4   B   Asthma

5   G   Pneumonia

Motor neurone disease causes muscle weakness. Wheeze and breathlessness with no fever are a good description of asthma. The fever and pleuritic chest pain are pathognomonic of pneumonia.

2.30 Infections

1	C	Cytomegalovirus
2	G	Respiratory syncytial virus
3	H	*Streptococcus pneumoniae*
4	E	*Mycobacterium tuberculosis*
5	F	*Pneumocystis carinii*

In the immunocompromised, cytomegalovirus is a common causative organism. The most common cause of pneumonia in children under the age of 1 year is respiratory syncytial virus. In adults the most common cause is *Streptococcus pneumoniae*. In drug addicts and people with HIV infection *Pneumocystis carinii* is common.

2.31 Endocrine Conditions

1	C	Cushing disease
2	D	Diabetes insipidus
3	A	Acromegaly
4	H	Prolactinoma
5	G	Hypothyroidism

Patients with bipolar syndrome are treated with lithium, and this has a tendency to cause diabetes insipidus. Acromegaly is diagnosed by an oral glucose tolerance test. Galactorrhoea is indicative of prolactinoma.

2.32 Severe Infections

1	E	Meningococcal septicaemia

2	F	Osteomyelitis

3	J	Pyelonephritis

4	C	Infective endocarditis

5	G	Peritonitis

Pyelonephritis can be differentiated from cystitis, as the patient has loin pain. Laparoscopic abdominal surgery is associated with a risk of perforation of the gut, leading to peritonitis.

2.33 Lower-limb Problems

1	C	Deep vein thrombosis

2	D	Dependent oedema

3	B	Congestive cardiac failure

4	G	Nephritic syndrome

5	A	Cellulitis

Women who are pregnant may have difficulty with mobility, and are susceptible to deep vein thrombosis. In Q 5 the clue is that the patient has been bitten by an insect, the overlying skin is red and painful, and he is diabetic, and therefore susceptible to infection.

2.34 Pre-operative Investigations

1 I Full blood count

2 D Coagulation screen

3 C Chest X-ray

4 B Cervical spine X-ray

5 G ERCP

The smoker awaiting operation on his varicose veins has signs of lung cancer (finger clubbing). This should be investigated as soon as possible. Patients who have severe rheumatoid arthritis may need a cervical spine X-ray to see whether there is any weakness of the vertebrae, which in an extreme case may lead to damage of the spinal cord during intubation. A patient awaiting gall bladder surgery who develops jaundice and raised liver function tests should be investigated by ERCP, which will show the biliary tree and pancreatic ducts.

2.35 Infections of the Lung

1 F *Mycobacterium tuberculosis*

2 D *Legionella pneumophila*

3 H *Pneumocystis carinii*

4 B Cytomegalovirus

5 I *Pseudomonas aeruginosa*

It is important to have an idea of which bacteria/viruses are prevalent in which age group and in different epidemiological categories. Hotels or places with poor air-conditioning systems are at risk of *Legionella* outbreaks. In patients with HIV infection, *Pneumocystis carinii* is the most common bacterium. Patients with cystic fibrosis are at risk of nasty pneumonias which can cause cavitation, such as pneumonia caused by *Pseudomonas*.

2.36 Tests

| 1 | F | Plasma glucose |

| 2 | I | Thyroxine (T4) |

| 3 | A | Alkaline phosphatase |

| 4 | D | Calcium |

| 5 | B | Amylase |

A patient with tachycardia and atrial fibrillation should be suspected of being hyperthyroid. Alkaline phosphatase is a marker for bony tumours. A patient with 'bones, stones, abdominal groans and psychic moans' should be suspected of having hypercalcaemia, usually secondary to primary hyperparathyroidism. Alcoholics with severe central abdominal pain should be suspected of having pancreatitis, and amylase is a marker for this.

3 Oral Medicine

3.1 Theme: Cranial Nerves
3.2 Theme: Headache
3.3 Theme: Neck Lumps
3.4 Theme: Oral Cavity Conditions
3.5 Theme: Painful Mouth
3.6 Theme: Viruses Causing Oral Lesions
3.7 Theme: Oral Drug Reactions
3.8 Theme: Oral Leukoplakia
3.9 Theme: Pemphigus
3.10 Theme: Benign Mucous Membrane Pemphigoid
3.11 Theme: Impetigo
3.12 Theme: Primary Syphilis
3.13 Theme: Herpes
3.14 Theme: Addison's Disease
3.15 Theme: Sjögren Syndrome
3.16 Theme: Trigeminal Neuralgia
3.17 Theme: Temporal Arteritis
3.18 Theme: Erythema Migrans
3.19 Theme: Median Rhomboid Glossitis
3.20 Theme: Orofacial Granulomatosis
3.21 Theme: Aphthous Ulceration (1)
3.22 Theme: Aphthous Ulceration (2)
3.23 Theme: Lichen Planus
3.24 Theme: Oral Manifestations of Endocrine Disease
3.25 Theme: Burning Mouth Syndrome
3.26 Theme: Eponymous Syndromes (1)
3.27 Theme: Eponymous Syndromes (2)
3.28 Theme: Paget's Disease

ORAL MEDICINE

3.1 Theme: Cranial Nerves

A	I	F	VI
B	II	G	VII
C	III	H	VIII
D	IV	I	IX and X
E	V	J	XII

For the following clinical scenarios, choose the most appropriate cranial nerve from the list above. Each option may be used once, more than once or not at all.

1. Bell's palsy is a lower motor neurone condition of this nerve.
2. Furosemide (Frusemide) may affect this nerve.
3. Lesion will lead to diplopia on lateral gaze.
4. Needed for the gag reflex.
5. The tongue will deviate to the side affected.

3.2 Theme: Headache

A	Cluster
B	Meningitis
C	Migraine
D	Post-herpetic neuralgia
E	Sinusitis
F	Temporal arteritis
G	Tension
H	Trigeminal neuralgia

For each of the following statements, choose the most closely associated diagnosis from the list above. You may use each option once, more than once or not at all.

1. C-reactive protein (CRP) levels may be used to monitor this condition.
2. Ergot medication can be used to treat this condition.
3. Most common cause of a headache.
4. Fever, photophobia, neck stiffness and rash.
5. Stabbing, intense pain lasting seconds on the face.

3.3 Theme: Neck Lumps

A Dermoid cyst
B Lymph nodes
C Parotid salivary calculus
D Submandibular salivary calculus
E Mandibular torus
F Thyroid nodule
G Thyroglossal cyst
H Torus palatinus

For each of the following clinical scenarios, choose the most appropriate diagnosis from the list above. You may use each option once, more than once or not at all.

1. If persistently enlarged neoplasia, needs to be excluded.
2. Lump moves on protraction of tongue.
3. Multiple congenital anomalies occurring in the midline.
4. Painful swelling at angle of mandible made worse on eating.
5. Sublingual swelling made worse on eating.

3.4 Theme: Oral Cavity Conditions

A *Candida*
B Fordyce spots
C Geographic tongue
D Leukoplakia
E Median rhomboid glossitis
F Necrotising ulcerative gingivitis
G Pellagra
H Scurvy

For each of the following statements, choose the most appropriate disease/condition from the list above. You may use each option once, more than once or not at all.

1. A smoker, male aged 19 years old complaining of very painful gums.
2. Deeply fissured tongue.
3. Erythema migrans linguae.
4. Smooth and red lips, glossitis with risk of developing dementia.
5. Up to 5% of this condition may become malignant.

3.5 Theme: Painful Mouth

A Acute necrotising ulcerative gingivitis (ANUG)
B Aphthous ulcer
C *Candida*
D Geographic tongue
E Leukoplakia
F Lichen planus
G Polyp
H Torus

For each of the following statements, choose the most appropriate diagnosis from the list above. You may use each option once, more than once or not at all.

1 Adjacent to a sanitary pontic on a bridge.
2 De-epithelialised area on mucosa.
3 Punched-out interdental papillae.
4 Over extended denture flange.
5 Removal of white membrane reveals a red area.

3.6 Theme: Viruses Causing Oral Lesions

A Coxsackie A
B Coxsackie B
C Cytomegalovirus
D Epstein–Barr
E Herpes simple
F Paramyxovirus
G Varicella zoster

For each of the following statements, choose the most appropriate diagnosis from the list above. You may use each option once, more than once or not at all.

1 A 6-year-old systemically unwell child with bilateral parotid swelling and mildly raised serum amylase.
2 A 6-year-old boy develops shallow ulcers on the gingival and tongue with vesicles on the palms and soles. The disease is reported as an outbreak at his pre-school group. It resolves over 2 weeks.
3 An 80-year-old woman presents with a rash on her right chin and lip. She has vesicles and ulcers on the buccal gingival on the mandibular right quadrant and right-hand side of her tongue. Before the rash came, she had dysaesthesia of the mandibular right trigeminal nerve.

ORAL MEDICINE

3.7 Theme: Oral Drug Reactions

A Bendroflumethiazide
B Captopril
C Cyanide
D Felodipine
E Gold
F Hydrocortisone
G Lead
H Proguanil

For each of the following statements, choose the most appropriate option from the list above. You may use each option once, more than once or not at all.

1 A 35-year-old man presents with a grey pencil line on his gingival margins. He lives in a derelict factory.

2 A woman who has been on safari for a number of months presents with discoloration of the mucous membranes.

3 A man who recently started on calcium-channel blockers presents with gingival hypertrophy.

4 The above man has his medication changed and reports oral dysaesthesia, but on examination the mouth is normal.

3.8 Theme: Oral Leukoplakia

A Chronic hyperplastic candidosis
B Darier's disease
C Dyskeratosis congenita
D Frictional keratosis
E Leukoedema
F Lichenoid drug reaction
G Oral cancer
H Stomatitis nicotina
I Systemic lupus erythematosus
J Tylosis
K White spongy naevus

For each of the following statements, choose the most appropriate diagnosis from the list above. You may use each option once, more than once or not at all.

1 A 26-year-old woman starts taking the combined contraceptive pill. She notes a rash on both cheeks that is spreading over her nose, and intra-orally there are bilateral white buccal striations.

2 A 75-year-old pipe smoker comes to see you for a new set of dentures. On examining the palate, you note the classic appearance of dark, distended minor salivary gland opening on an erythematous background.

3 A congenital oral leukoplakia, which has no malignant potential.

ORAL MEDICINE

3.9 Theme: Pemphigus

A Male
B Female
C Equally prevalent in males and females
D Less than 24 hours
E 1-3 days
F 3-7 days
G Immunofluorescence
H Staining with methylene blue
I Staining with Ziehl-Nielsen stain
J Jones
K Nichols' sign
L Nikolsky's sign
M Swinton
N IgA
O IgG
P IgM
Q Do nothing, it spontaneously heals
R Excision
S Systemic corticosteroids
T Topical antibiotics

For each of the following questions, choose the most appropriate option from the list above. You may use each option once, more than once or not at all.

1. In which sex is pemphigus most prevalent?
2. How long do the lesions last before they rupture?
3. Which eponymous sign is diagnostic for this condition?
4. Which special test do you need to perform on the biopsy?
5. Which immunoglobulin is found binding to intercellular attachments?
6. How would you treat this condition?

3.10 Theme: Benign Mucous Membrane Pemphigoid

A   Male
B   Female
C   Equally prevalent in males and females
D   18–30 years
E   31–45 years
F   45–60 years
G   60+ years
H   Intra-epithelial
I   Subepithelial
J   Less than 24 hours
K   1–3 days
L   3–7 days
M   Desquamative gingivitis
N   Lichen planus
O   Oral cancer
P   Induration
Q   Retinopathy
R   Symblepharon

For each of the following questions, choose the most appropriate option from the list above. You may use each option once, more than once or not at all.

1   In which sex is the condition most prevalent?
2   In which age group is the disease most prevalent?
3   Is it a subepithelial or intra-epithelial lesion?
4   How long do the lesions last before they burst?
5   Which other oral condition is pemphigoid associated with?
6   What is the correct name for the ocular scarring that may lead to blindness?

ORAL MEDICINE

3.11 Theme: Impetigo

A Group A streptococcus
B *Streptococcus milleri*
C *Streptococcus mutans*
D *Treponema pallidum*
E Under 10 years
F 18–30 years
G 30–50 years
H 50+ years
I Amoxicillin
J Tetracycline
K Erythromycin
L Flucloxacillin
M Metronidazole
N Cancrum oris
O Necrotising fasciitis
P Toxic epidermal necrolysis
Q Social class I
R Social class II
S Social class III
T Social class IV
U Social class V

For each of the following questions, choose the most appropriate option from the list above. You may use each option once, more than once or not at all.

1. What is the main causative organism?
2. Which age group is this most commonly found in?
3. In which social class is it most prevalent?
4. Which is the systemic drug of choice?
5. What is the topical drug of choice?
6. In the rare cases which are caused by *Staphylococcus aureus*, what severe condition may it cause?

3.12 Theme: Primary Syphilis

A   *Borrelia burgdorferi*
B   *Shigella*
C   *Staphylococcus aureus*
D   *Treponema pallidum*
E   Floor of mouth
F   Lip
G   Palate
H   Tongue
I   1 week
J   1-3 months
K   3-6 months
L   1 year
M   Chancre
N   Gumma
O   Snail tracks
P   Culturing on chocolate agar
Q   Dark-field microscopy
R   Immunofluorescence
S   Excision
T   No treatment
U   Metronidazole
V   Penicillin

For each of the following questions, choose the most appropriate option from the list above. You may use each option once, more than once or not at all.

1   What is the causative organism?
2   Where is the lesion usually found?
3   What is the name of the primary lesion?
4   How long does the lesion last before it heals spontaneously?
5   Which blood test would you do to confirm the presence of the causative organism?
6   What is the treatment for this condition?

ORAL MEDICINE

3.13 Theme: Herpes

A	HHV 1	E	HHV 5
B	HHV 2	F	HHV 6
C	HHV 3	G	HHV 7
D	HHV 4	H	HHV 8

Match the correct name to the appropriate human herpesvirus (HHV).

1. Roseola infantum
2. Kaposi's sarcoma
3. Epstein-Barr virus
4. Herpetic whitlow
5. Zoster
6. Cytomegalovirus

3.14 Theme: Addison's Disease

A	Adrenal gland	M	Hyperpigmentation
B	Hypothalamus	N	T_4 blood test
C	Anterior pituitary	O	Thyroid stimulating hormone (TSH) test
D	Posterior pituitary		
E	Thyroid	P	Adrenocorticotropic hormone (ACTH) tolerance test
F	Thyroxine		
G	Corticosteroids	Q	Brown
H	Calcitrol	R	Red
I	Mineralocorticoids	S	White
J	Ulcers	T	Thyroxine
K	Raised polypoid lesions	U	Carbimazole
L	Lichenoid lesions		

For each of the following questions, choose the most appropriate option from the list above. You may use each option once, more than once or not at all.

1. Which gland is atrophic in Addison's disease?
2. What substance is low or absent in this condition?
3. What lesions are present on the gingivae and the skin?
4. What colour are these lesions?
5. How would you diagnose this condition?
6. How would you treat this condition?

3.15 Theme: Sjögren Syndrome

A	Swelling
B	Too much saliva
C	Xerostomia
D	Male
E	Female
F	Equally prevalent in males and females
G	Auto-antibodies
H	Sialography
I	Labial gland biopsy deep to muscle
J	18–30 years
K	30–50 years
L	50+ years
M	Osteoarthritis
N	Rheumatoid arthritis
O	Seronegative arthritis
P	Anti-muscarinic drugs
Q	Corticosteroids
R	Pilocarpine

For each of the following questions, choose the most appropriate option from the list above. You may use each option once, more than once or not at all.

1. What is the main oral complaint in this condition?
2. Which sex is more commonly affected by this disorder?
3. In which age group does it most commonly present?
4. How would you definitively diagnose this condition?
5. What other systemic condition is this condition associated with?
6. Which systemic drug can help to alleviate this condition?

ORAL MEDICINE

3.16 Theme: Trigeminal Neuralgia

A	18–30 years
B	30–50 years
C	50+ years
D	Male
E	Female
F	Equally prevalent in males and females
G	Constant
H	Dull
I	Sharp
J	Shooting
K	Dental abscess
L	Nothing
M	Trigger factor
N	Biopsy
O	Blood tests
P	Clinical history only
Q	Carbamazepine
R	Corticosteroids
S	Fluconazole
T	Phenytoin

For each of the following questions, choose the most appropriate option from the list above. You may use each option once, more than once or not at all.

1. In which age group is this condition most prevalent?
2. In which sex is this condition most prevalent?
3. What is the classic description of the pain associated with this condition?
4. What brings on the pain?
5. How do you diagnose the condition?
6. What is the drug of choice in this condition?

3.17 Theme: Temporal Arteritis

A 18–30 years
B 30–50 years
C 50+ years
D Male
E Female
F Affects males and females equally
G Paraesthesia
H Trismus
I Claudication
J Stroke
K Blindness
L Hypertension
M Full blood count
N Liver function tests
O Thyroxine levels
P Erythrocyte sedimentation rate (ESR)
Q Excision of the lesion
R Corticosteroids (high dose)
S Analgesia only

For each of the following questions, choose the most appropriate option from the list above. You may use each option once, more than once or not at all.

1 Which age group does this condition affect?
2 Which sex does it affect most commonly?
3 What extra-oral problem can occur in patients with this condition?
4 What is the major risk in this condition which makes it a medical emergency?
5 Which blood test helps confirm the diagnosis?
6 What is the treatment?

3.18 Theme: Erythema Migrans

A Lichen planus
B Lichenoid reaction
C Geographical tongue
D Scrotal tongue
E 1:1000
F 1%
G 10%
H 20%
I Rheumatoid arthritis
J Osteoarthritis
K Psoriasis
L Hot foods
M Acidic foods
N Cold food
O Irregular red de-papillation
P White lacy striae bilaterally
Q Regular white de-papillation
R White raised lesion
S Reassure the patient, no treatment
T Biopsy with immunofluorescence
U Excision
V Corticosteroids

For each of the following questions, choose the most appropriate option from the list above. You may use each option once, more than once or not at all.

1. What is the most common name of this condition?
2. How prevalent is this condition in the population?
3. What other condition is it associated with?
4. What type of food makes it painful?
5. What can be seen in the areas affected by the condition?
6. How do you treat this condition?

ORAL MEDICINE

3.19 Theme: Median Rhomboid Glossitis

A 18–30 years
B 30–45 years
C 45–60 years
D 60+ years
E Male
F Female
G Equally prevalent in males and females
H *Staphylococcus aureus*
I *Streptococcus*
J *Treponema*
K *Candida albicans*
L Alcoholism
M Drug taking
N Smoking
O Anorexia
P Flucloxacillin
Q Metronidazole
R Fluconazole
S Leukaemia
T HIV
U Tuberculosis

For each of the following questions, choose the most appropriate option from the list above. You may use each option once, more than once or not at all.

1. In which age group is median rhomboid glossitis most prevalent?
2. In which sex is this condition most prevalent?
3. Which organism is associated with the condition?
4. Which habit is associated with this condition?
5. How do you treat this condition?
6. Which systemic condition is associated with this lesion, if it occurs in a younger person?

3.20 Theme: Orofacial Granulomatosis

A　Male
B　Female
C　Equally prevalent in males and females
D　Under 18 years
E　18-30 years
F　30-50 years
G　50+ years
H　African-Caribbean
I　Asian
J　White
K　Coeliac disease
L　Crohn's disease
M　Diverticulitis
N　Gardner syndrome
O　Melkersson–Rosenthal syndrome
P　Peutz–Jeghers syndrome
Q　Intralesional corticosteroids
R　Nothing, it will decrease in size with time
S　Systemic corticosteroids

For each of the following questions, choose the most appropriate option from the list above. You may use each option once, more than once or not at all.

1　In which sex is orofacial granulomatosis most prevalent?
2　In which age group is this condition most prevalent?
3　In which ethnic group is this condition most prevalent?
4　Which systemic condition is it most commonly associated with?
5　In which syndrome is the facial swelling associated with a fissured tongue and a facial palsy?
6　What is the correct treatment for it?

ORAL MEDICINE

3.21 Theme: Aphthous Ulceration (1)

A	Under 18 years	I	5%
B	18-30 years	J	25%
C	30-50 years	K	40%
D	50+ years	L	50%
E	Male	M	1 mm
F	Female	N	2-5 mm
G	Male and females equally affected	O	5+ mm
H	1%		

For each of the following questions, choose the most appropriate option from the list above. You may use each option once, more than once or not at all.

1. In which age group does aphthous ulceration initially present?
2. In which sex is aphthous ulceration most prevalent?
3. What proportion of the population is affected by aphthous ulceration?
4. What size are minor aphthous ulcers?
5. What size are major aphthous ulcers?
6. What size are herpetiform aphthous ulcers?

3.22 Theme: Aphthous Ulceration (2)

A	Less than 5
B	5-14 days
C	Less than 10
D	14-31 days
E	10-30
F	31-60 days
G	30+

For each of the following questions, choose the most appropriate option from the list above. You may use each option once, more than once or not at all.

1. How many minor aphthous ulcers are usually present?
2. How many major aphthous ulcers are usually present?
3. How many herpetiform aphthous ulcers are usually present?
4. How long do minor aphthous ulcers take to heal?
5. How long do major aphthous ulcers take to heal?
6. How long do minor herpetiform ulcers take to heal?

ORAL MEDICINE

3.23 Theme: Lichen Planus

A	Under 18 years
B	18–30 years
C	30–50 years
D	50+ years
E	Male
F	Female
G	Equally prevalent among men and women
H	Atrophic
I	Erosive
J	Papular
K	Reticular
L	Bence Jones lesions
M	Caldwell spots
N	Wickham's striae
O	Back
P	Extensor surfaces of the arms
Q	Face
R	Flexor surfaces of the arms
S	Biopsy
T	Blood tests
U	Clinical assessment only
V	Virology

For each of the following questions, choose the most appropriate option from the list above. You may use each option once, more than once or not at all.

1. In which age group does lichen planus most commonly present?
2. Which sex is affected most by this condition?
3. Which type of lichen planus has the greatest malignant potential?
4. What is the name of the cutaneous lesions of lichen planus?
5. Where are they found?
6. How do you diagnose lichen planus?

3.24 Theme: Oral Manifestations of Endocrine Disease

A	Acromegaly
B	Addison's disease
C	Cushing syndrome
D	Diabetes
E	Hyperparathyroidism
F	Hyperthyroidism
G	Hypoparathyroidism
H	Hypothyroidism
I	Sex hormones

For each of the following oral manifestations, choose the most appropriate endocrine disease option from the list above. You may use each option once, more than once or not at all.

1 Enlargement of the lips and tongue, spacing of the teeth, and an increase in jaw size, particularly the mandible, resulting in a Class III malocclusion.

2 Melanotic brown hyperpigmentation of the oral mucosa, commonly the cheek.

3 The appearance of a 'moon face' and oral candidosis.

4 The congenital form of this disease is associated with puffy enlargement of the lips and delayed tooth eruption.

5 Increased susceptibility to periodontal disease, xerostomia. Some patients with this condition complain of oral dysaesthesia.

6 This endocrine disorder causes radiographic changes in the mandible. It causes the loss of the lamina dura, a 'ground glass' appearance of bone and cystic lesions which are indistinguishable from a 'Brown's tumour'.

ORAL MEDICINE

3.25 Theme: Burning Mouth Syndrome

A	Male
B	Female
C	Equally prevalent in men and women
D	18–30 years
E	30–45 years
F	45–60 years
G	60+ years
H	Floor of mouth
I	Lips
J	Palate
K	Pharynx
L	Tongue
M	Crohn's disease
N	Diabetes
O	HIV
P	Vitamin A
Q	Vitamin B_6
R	Vitamin B_{12}
S	Vitamin E
T	*Candida albicans*
U	*Staphylococcus aureus*
V	*Streptococcus pyogenes*

For each of the following questions, choose the most appropriate option from the list above. You may use each option once, more than once or not at all.

1. Which sex is mainly affected with burning mouth syndrome?
2. In which age group does this condition first present?
3. Which site is most commonly affected with the condition?
4. Which systemic condition must be ruled out in patients with burning mouth syndrome?
5. Which vitamin is most commonly low in these patients?
6. Which bacteria are commonly associated with this condition?

3.26 Theme: Eponymous Syndromes (1)

A   Albright syndrome
B   Behçet syndrome
C   Crouzon syndrome
D   Ehlers Danlos syndrome
E   Frey syndrome
F   Gardner syndrome
G   Graves' disease
H   Horner syndrome
I   Larsen syndrome
J   Melkersson–Rosenthal syndrome

For each of the following descriptions, choose the most appropriate disorder from the list above. You may use each option once, more than once or not at all.

1   Classically a picture of oral ulceration, genital ulceration and uveitis. Clinical diagnosis can be made on finding two of these three. It is a multisystem disease of immunological origin. It tends to affect young adults, especially males, and there is an association with HLA-B5. It undergoes spontaneous remission.

2   This comprises a group of disorders characterised by hyper-flexibility of joints, increased bleeding and bruising, and hyper-extensible skin. There appears to be an underlying molecular abnormality of collagen.

3   This syndrome consists of facial paralysis, facial oedema and a fissured tongue. It is a variant of orofacial granulomatosis.

4   Consists of a constricted pupil (miosis), drooping eyelid (ptosis), and unilateral loss of sweating (anhydrosis) on the face and occasionally enophthalmos. It is caused by an interruption of the sympathetic nerve at the cervical ganglion secondary to a tumour.

5   A condition in which gustatory sweating and flushing of the skin occurs. It follows trauma to the salivary glands and is thought to be caused by crossover of the sympathetic and parasympathetic innervation to the gland and the skin.

6   Auto-antibodies to thyroid-stimulating hormone (TSH) cause hyperthyroidism with ophthalmopathy.

ORAL MEDICINE

3.27 Theme: Eponymous Syndromes (2)

A   Apert syndrome
B   Chediak–Higashi syndrome
C   Down syndrome
D   Gorlin–Goltz syndrome
E   Hurler syndrome
F   Patterson–Brown–Kelly syndrome (Plummer–Vinson)
G   Progeria
H   Ramsay–Hunt syndrome
I   Stevens–Johnson syndrome
J   Sturge–Weber anomalad
K   Von Recklinghausen syndrome

For each of the following descriptions, choose the most appropriate disorder from the list above. You may use each option once, more than once or not at all.

1. The commonest of malformation syndromes caused by trisomy of chromosome 21. The patient has macroglossia, delayed eruption of teeth, small nose, brachycephaly, midface retrusion and upward-sloping palpebral fissures.

2. Multiple neurofibromas with skin pigmentation, skeletal abnormalities, central nervous syndrome involvement, and a predisposition to malignancy. Autosomal dominant.

3. A severe version of erythema multiforme, a mucocutaneous disorder, probably autoimmune in nature and precipitated classically by drugs. Classical lesions are target lesions, concentric red rings which especially affect the hands and feet.

4. A lower-motor neurone facial palsy with vesicles on the same side in the pharynx, external auditory canal and on the face. May lead to deafness. Caused by herpes zoster.

5. The occurrence of dysphagia, microcytic hypochromic anaemia, koilonychia (spoon shaped nails), and angular cheilitis. The dysphagia is due to a post-cricoid web, usually a membrane on the anterior oesophageal wall, which is premalignant. Affects mainly middle-aged women.

6. Consists of multiple basal cell naevi, multiple odontogenic keratocysts, calcified falx cerebri, cleidocranial dysostosis.

ORAL MEDICINE

3.28 Theme: Paget's Disease

A   18-30 years
B   30-50 years
C   50+ years
D   Herpes
E   HIV
F   Measles
G   Mumps
H   Mandible
I   Maxilla
J   External resorption
K   Hypercementosis
L   Increased cystic formation
M   Periodontal disease
N   Cotton wool
O   Ground glass
P   Sunray
Q   Alanine aminotransferase
R   Alkaline phosphatase
S   Bilirubin

For each of the following questions, choose the most appropriate option from the list above. You may use each option once, more than once or not at all.

1. Which age group is affected by Paget's disease?
2. Which virus has been implicated in the aetiology of this disease?
3. Is the mandible or maxilla most frequently affected?
4. How does it affect the teeth?
5. What is the classic description of the radiological appearance of the bone?
6. Which biochemical marker is raised in this condition?

116 ORAL MEDICINE

ANSWERS

3.1 Cranial Nerves

1 G VII

2 H VIII

3 F VI

4 I IX and X

5 J XII

Furosemide has been reported to be ototoxic due to possible effects on the vestibulocochlear (auditory) cranial nerve. Cranial nerve VII is the facial nerve and is mainly motor. The sixth cranial nerve is the abducens; complete interruption of the peripheral sixth nerve causes diplopia (double vision), due to the unopposed action of the medial rectus muscle. Glossopharyngeal IX and vagus X nerves are considered together because they exit from the brain stem side by side. The gag reflex has a sensory and a motor limb. The sensory limb is mediated predominantly by cranial nerve IX, while the motor limb by cranial nerve X. The XII is the hypoglossal cranial nerve and, if damaged, deviation of the tongue towards the paralysed side will occur when the tongue is stuck out.

3.2 Headache

1 F Temporal arteritis

2 C Migraine

3 G Tension

4 B Meningitis

5 H Trigeminal neuralgia

Cluster headaches are excruciating attacks of pain in one side of the head, often felt around the eye.

Post-herpetic neuralgia is a nerve pain due to damage caused by the varicella zoster virus. Typically, the neuralgia is confined to a dermatomic area of the skin and follows an outbreak of herpes zoster (commonly known as 'shingles') in that same dermatomic area.

Sinusitis is an infection of a sinus such as maxillary or frontal frequently following a head cold. Tenderness is usually present over the sinus affected.

3.3 Neck Lumps

1 B Lymph nodes

2 G Thyroglossal cyst

3 A Dermoid cyst

4 C Parotid salivary calculus

5 D Submandibular salivary calculus

Persistent swollen lymph nodes may be associated with metastatic disease and need investigation.

Mandibular tori are usually on the lingual aspect close to the premolars. They are bony growths and normal for some individuals. A torus palatinus similarly is normal for some individuals occurring on the middle of the palate.

Thyroid nodules are neoplasms usually; they are frequently benign but need investigation.

Often parotid swelling is unilateral; if it is bilateral, other infective diseases such as mumps should be considered. If it is unilateral, it is most likely to either be an obstruction of the gland or infective (ie sialadenitis). The swelling is more common at mealtimes when the gland produces saliva and this is unable to flow through the gland.

Dermoid cysts can be found in all areas of the body, and the location often depends on the contents of the cyst. They are thin-walled tumours that contain different amounts of fat and other substances.

Sublingual swellings that are worse on eating are more likely to be associated with the salivary gland as opposed to a ranula.

3.4 Oral Cavity Conditions

| 1 | F | Necrotising ulcerative gingivitis |

| 2 | C | Geographic tongue |

| 3 | C | Geographic tongue |

| 4 | G | Pellagra |

| 5 | D | Leukoplakia |

Fordyce spots are visible sebaceous glands that are present in most individuals.

Median rhomboid glossitis or glossal central papillary atrophy is a condition characterised by an area of redness and loss of lingual papillae, situated on the dorsum of the tongue in the midline immediately in front of the circumvallate papillae. The cause is usually a chronic candidal infection.

Pellagra is due to vitamin B_3 (niacin) deficiency. It is rare in the UK but can result from alcoholism or malabsorption. Often patients develop changes in mood or personality associated with weakness and loss of appetite.

Scurvy is due to vitamin C deficiency. It is rare in the UK but may be seen in some elderly people or those with unusual diets. Common features are purpura and dermatitis. In advanced disease poor healing and swollen bleeding gums are evidence.

Necrotising ulcerative gingivitis is more common in young males, who often are smokers with neglected mouths. It is important to exclude any underlying systemic disease or immunosuppression in such patients.

Leukoplakia is defined as a white patch which cannot be wiped off the mucosa or be diagnosed with any other disease process. There is often no specific appearance, but it is tough and has a plaque-like appearance within the soft tissues, usually irregular. Most show no dysplasia histologically; however, there are some which do, therefore biopsy is important to confirm the diagnosis.

ORAL MEDICINE

3.5 Painful Mouth

1 G Polyp

2 B Aphthous ulcer

3 A ANUG

4 G Polyp

5 C *Candida*

Fibrous lesions in the mouth are very common. Fibro-epithelial polyps are frequently caused by trauma and are hyperplastic swellings, also caused by low-grade infection. Sanitary pontics have a gap between the bridge and ridge. Many individuals suck their cheek or tongue through the gap and develop polyps. Similarly, denture flanges, particularly if over-extended, can cause polyps.

Punched-out interdental papillae are characteristic of cases of ANUG. Often they can 'slough' away as well with a very distinctive odour.

Apthous ulceration (recurrent aphthous stomatitis) is one of the commonest mucosal diseases in the oral cavity. It can be due to a variety of causes, usually trauma. It can be minor, major or herpetiform. Usually a single isolated traumatic ulcer heals within 1–2 weeks. It is important to exclude any other causes for the ulceration.

A torus is a bony lump usually on the palate or lingually next to the premolars. Tori are normal for some individuals and are usually left in situ.

Lichen planus is a chronic inflammatory disease that can affect the skin and mucous membranes. The classical appearance is that of 'striae' in the mucous membrane or a lacy pattern. Lesions are often symmetrical and bilateral particularly in the buccal mucosa, but can present anywhere in the oral cavity. Patients may have associated cutaneous lesions, particularly on the flexor surfaces of joint. Lichen planus can also be found on mucous membranes in the genital regions and ocular areas.

Candida can cause a variety of diseases, either acute or chronic. It forms soft, creamy like plaques on the oral mucosa. Distinctively, it can be wiped off, unlike other pathologies such as lichen planus or a leukoplakia.

Leukoplakia is a white patch that is usually a keratosis and cannot be removed by rubbing, unlike *Candida* infections.

3.6 Viruses Causing Oral Lesions

1 F Paramyxovirus

This child has mumps.

2 A Coxsackie A

This child has hand, foot and mouth disease.

3 G Varicella zoster

This woman has shingles of the mandibular division of the trigeminal nerve.

3.7 Oral Drug Reactions

1 G Lead

Lead poisoning produces a pencil line deposition in the tissues.

2 H Proguanil

This woman has been taking antimalarial drugs.

3 D Felodipine

Calcium-channel blockers, ie nifedipine, and anti-epileptics, ie phenytoin, cause gingival hyperplasia.

4 B Captopril

Angiotensin-converting enzyme (ACE) inhibitors can be associated with oral dysaesthesia.

ORAL MEDICINE

3.8 Oral Leukoplakia

1 I Systemic lupus erythematosus (SLE)

SLE can present after a new medication and presents with butterfly rash.

2 H Stomatitis nicotina

This is the description of stomatitis nicotina.

3 K White spongy naevus

This has no malignant potential.

3.9 Pemphigus

1 B Female

2 D Less than 24 hours

3 L Nikolsky's sign

4 G Immunofluorescence

5 O IgG

6 S Systemic corticosteroids

Pemphigus is an autoimmune disorder which affects females more than males. It is particularly prevalent in middle-aged Mediterranean women. The oral lesions are more prevalent and often precede the skin lesions. The bullae are fragile and burst within 24 hours, leaving painful ragged ulcers. Nikolsky's sign is diagnostic: digital pressure on the mucosa produces a bulla. The biopsy is studied under immunofluorescence and it shows IgG and C3 bound to intercellular attachments of epithelial cells. Pemphigus is treated with systemic corticosteroids.

3.10 Benign Mucous Membrane Pemphigoid

1 B Female

2 G 60+ years

3 I Subepithelial

4 K 1–3 days

5 M Desquamative gingivitis

6 R Symblepharon

Benign mucous pemphigoid is a condition which is more prevalent in women than men. It tends to occur in people over 60 years of age. The blood blisters are more durable than those of pemphigus and tend to last 1–3 days before they burst. The ulcers heal with scarring. Scarring in the larynx can lead to stenosis, and scarring in the conjunctiva can lead to symblepharon and blindness. The biopsy should be studied under immunofluorescence to show IgG and the subepithelial splitting. Treatment is with corticosteroids.

ORAL MEDICINE

3.11 Impetigo

1 A Group A streptococcus

2 E Under 10 years

3 U Social class V

4 L Flucloxacillin

5 J Tetracycline

6 P Toxic epidermal necrolysis

Impetigo is a condition caused by group A streptococcus, and mainly occurs in underprivileged children. It is highly contagious. Papules change into vesicles surrounded by erythema, and then into pustules with a golden crust. In rare cases where the cause is *Staphylococcus aureus* it can lead to toxic epidermal necrolysis.

3.12 Primary Syphilis

1 D *Treponema pallidum*

2 H Tongue

3 M Chancre

4 J 1–3 months

5 Q Dark-field microscopy

6 V Penicillin

Primary syphilis is caused by *Treponema pallidum*, and this is viewed under dark-field microscopy. It occurs mainly on the tongue as a central punched out ulcer known as a chancre. Primary syphilis is treated with penicillin.

3.13 Herpes

1	F	HHV 6
2	H	HHV 8
3	D	HHV 4
4	A	HHV 1
5	C	HHV 3
6	E	HHV 5

- Human herpesvirus 1 – herpetic infection 'above the waist'
- Human herpesvirus 2 – herpetic infection 'below the waist'
- Human herpesvirus 3 – varicella zoster, chicken pox or the recurrence shingles
- Human herpesvirus 4 – Epstein–Barr virus, more commonly known as glandular fever
- Human herpesvirus 5 – Cytomegalovirus
- Human herpesvirus 6 – Roseola infantum (red baby syndrome)
- Human herpesvirus 7 – 'mono-like' illness, pityriasis rosea
- Human herpesvirus 8 – Associated with Kaposi's sarcoma

ORAL MEDICINE

3.14 Addison's Disease

1 A Adrenal gland

2 G Corticosteroids

3 M Hyperpigmentation

4 Q Brown

5 P ACTH tolerance test

6 G Corticosteroids

Addison's disease is caused by adrenocortical atrophy or destruction of the adrenal gland. It mainly occurs when patients are being treated for long periods with systemic steroids, leading to the atrophy of the gland. There is brown pigmentation of the gingivae and the skin. Diagnosis is with the Synacthen test (response to ACTH). Treatment is with corticosteroids. Patients on long-term steroids require steroid cover for dental treatment to prevent an addisonian crisis.

3.15 Sjögren Syndrome

1 C Xerostomia

2 E Female

3 K 30–50 years

4 I Labial gland biopsy deep to muscle

5 N Rheumatoid arthritis

6 R Pilocarpine

Sjögren syndrome is an autoimmune condition that occurs mainly in middle-aged women. It causes dry mouth, dry eyes and dry genitals. There is increased root caries and problems with taste. The definitive diagnosis is with a labial gland biopsy deep to muscle. Sialography and the presence of auto-antibodies may help to confirm the diagnosis, but these are not definitive. Treatment is with pilocarpine and saliva substitutes.

3.16 Trigeminal Neuralgia

1 C 50+ years

2 F Equally prevalent in males and females

3 J Shooting

4 M Trigger factor

5 P Clinical history only

6 Q Carbamazepine

Trigeminal neuralgia is an excruciating condition affecting people over 50. It presents as an electric shock-like pain of rapid and short onset. It may be brought on by a trigger such as cold water, shaving or pressure. Diagnosis is by history alone. It is treated effectively with carbamazepine as long as there is good patient compliance. Patients need to have their liver function tested and full blood count checked when they are on this medicine, as it can cause an aplastic anaemia and derangement of liver function.

3.17 Temporal Arteritis

1 C 50+ years

2 F Affects males and females equally

3 I Claudication

4 K Blindness

5 P ESR

6 R Corticosteroids (high dose)

Temporal arteritis is a condition that occurs in older age groups. The pain is localised to the temporal and frontal region and usually described as a severe ache. The affected area is tender to touch. The major risk is involvement of the retinal arteries with sudden loss of vision. The underlying pathology is inflammatory arteritis. The diagnosis is made on the basis of the classic distribution of pain, the presence of jaw claudication and a raised ESR. The treatment is systemic steroids.

3.18 Erythema Migrans

1 C Geographical tongue

2 F 1%

3 K Psoriasis

4 M Acidic foods

5 O Irregular red de-papillation

6 S Reassure the patient, no treatment

Geographical tongue is a common condition associated with psoriasis. It occurs in 1–2% of the population and presents with areas of irregular, red depapillation. These red areas change in shape, increase in size and spread or move to other areas within hours. The condition typically involves the dorsum of the tongue, rarely the adjacent mucosa. The tongue is often fissured. Reassure the patient, as there is no treatment for this condition.

3.19 Median Rhomboid Glossitis

1　C　45-60 years

2　E　Male

3　K　*Candida albicans*

4　N　Smoking

5　R　Fluconazole

6　T　HIV

Median rhomboid glossitis occurs mainly in middle-aged men who smoke. It is associated with candidal infection. Suspect HIV infection, if this occurs in younger age groups.

3.20 Orofacial Granulomatosis

1　B　Female

2　D　Under 18 years

3　H　African-Caribbean

4　L　Crohn's disease

5　O　Melkersson-Rosenthal

6　Q　Intralesional corticosteroids

Orofacial granulomatosis is associated with Crohn's disease, and occurs in African-Caribbean females under 18 years of age. It is treated with intralesional steroids and is occasionally excised.

3.21 Aphthous Ulceration (1)

1	A	Under 18 years
2	F	Female
3	J	25%
4	N	2-5 mm
5	O	5+ mm
6	M	1 mm

Recurrent aphthous ulceration initially presents in the under-18 age group. It affects females more commonly than males. It is usually a life-long condition, but there can be long periods without ulceration. It is heavily linked to stress and dietary deficiency, besides having other risk factors.

3.22 Aphthous Ulceration (2)

1 C Less than 10

2 A Less than 5

3 G 30+

4 B 5-14 days

5 F 31-60 days

6 D 14-31 days

There are three different types of recurrent aphthous stomatitis:

- Minor – which first presents in the under-18s but tends to be life-long. The ulcers are less than 5 mm in diameter, classically heal within 14 days and heal without scarring.
- Major – involves large ulceration of greater than 10 mm in size. Classically there are greater than 10, but there can be less than 10. They can occur on any site, including the dorsum of the tongue and the palate. They can take up to 2 months to heal, and heal with scarring.
- Herpetiform – involves multiple minute ulcers that coalesce to produce large ragged ulcers. Initially there are between 30 to 100 vesicles which produce the large ulceration. They can take up to a month to heal.

There is a mnemonic for the risk factors for recurrent aphthous stomatitis (for the not easily offended): DEAP SH*T.

- Deficiency – iron, folate or B_{12}
- Endocrine – women seem to find that the ulceration tends to occur in the luteal phase of their menstrual cycle
- Allergy – a change in toothpaste or mouthwash may precipitate a bout of ulceration
- Psychological – stress is a major risk factor. Teenagers tend to present with their first bout of ulceration during important examinations
- Smoking – smoking is a risk factor
- Hereditary – there is a familial link, especially in twins
- Immunological – there is ongoing research into the presence of specific immunoglobulins involved in the production of aphthae

ORAL MEDICINE

- Trauma – minor trauma such as lip biting, or minor burns with hot food have been implicated.

Management involves treating any underlying predisposing factors. Adcortyl in Orabase has been suggested as being efficacious in the treatment of aphthae. Some find it more beneficial than others.

3.23 Lichen Planus

| 1 | C | 30–50 years |

| 2 | F | Female |

| 3 | I | Erosive |

| 4 | J | Papular |

| 5 | R | Flexor surfaces of the arms |

| 6 | S | Biopsy |

Lichen planus is a mucocutaneous disorder. The aetiology is unknown. Either the skin lesions or the mucosal lesions can be involved on their own, but most commonly they are found together. It usually presents as bilateral white lacy striae in the buccal mucosa. The most common type is the reticular form, but there are many forms, including plaque-like, atrophic, reticular, papular, erosive and bullous. The skin lesions mainly affect the flexor arms but may also affect the shins. The cutaneous lesions are pink/purple papules. Patients complain that hot and spicy foods irritate the lesions and are painful. This condition can be treated with Adcortyl in Orabase. The lesions must be biopsied to differentiate them from other lesions, especially lichenoid reaction and cancer. Mystifyingly, lichen planus often spontaneously resolves on its own.

3.24 Oral Manifestations of Endocrine Disease

1 A Acromegaly

2 B Addison's disease

3 C Cushing syndrome

4 H Hypothyroidism

5 D Diabetes

6 E Hyperparathyroidism

It is important to recognise orofacial manifestations of endocrine diseases as these are quite prevalent in the population.

3.25 Burning Mouth Syndrome

1 B Female

2 G 60+ years

3 L Tongue

4 N Diabetes

5 R Vitamin B_{12}

6 T *Candida albicans*

Burning mouth syndrome is seven times as likely to affect women as men. There are many risk factors and it is important to rule out medical causes before investigating psychological causes. The main medical causes are iron, folate and vitamin B_{12} deficiency, and diabetes mellitus. Allergy to denture bases, toothpaste and poorly constructed dentures are other causes. Psychological causes are stress, depression, cancerphobia and the onset of the menopause.

ORAL MEDICINE

3.26 Eponymous Syndromes (1)

1 B Behçet syndrome

2 D Ehlers Danlos syndrome

3 J Melkersson-Rosenthal syndrome

4 H Horner syndrome

5 E Frey syndrome

6 G Graves' disease

There are many groups of syndromes which are *viva* favourites. It is important to learn them as they also often come up in written papers.

3.27 Eponymous Syndromes (2)

1 C Down syndrome

2 K Von Recklinghausen syndrome

3 I Stevens-Johnson syndrome

4 H Ramsay-Hunt syndrome

5 F Patterson-Brown-Kelly syndrome (Plummer-Vinson)

6 D Gorlin-Goltz syndrome

There are many groups of syndromes, especially those which encompass autoimmune conditions.

ORAL MEDICINE

3.28 Paget's Disease

1 C 50+ years

2 F Measles

3 I Maxilla

4 K Hypercementosis

5 N Cotton wool

6 R Alkaline phosphatase

Paget's disease commonly affects the over-50s. It affects the skull, long bones and pelvis, as well as the jaws. The aetiology is unknown, although measles and respiratory syncytial virus (RSV) have been implicated. The maxilla is most frequently affected. Hypercementosis affects the roots of the teeth and makes extraction difficult. There is a replacement of normal bone by a chaotic alternation of resorption and deposition, with resorption dominating in the early stages. Bone pain and neuropathy are common. The radiographs show a 'cotton wool' appearance. Biochemistry shows raised alkaline phosphatase. Avoid general anaesthetic and plan extractions surgically. Diphosphonates and calcitonin are used in treatment.

4 Oral Pathology

- 4.1 Theme: Autoantibodies/Autoimmune Diseases
- 4.2 Theme: Cranial Nerves
- 4.3 Theme: Peripheral Nerve Injuries
- 4.4 Theme: Skin Infections
- 4.5 Theme: Systemic Conditions Associated with Root Resorption
- 4.6 Theme: Eponymous Syndromes
- 4.7 Theme: Oral 'Lumps and Bumps'
- 4.8 Theme: Oropharyngeal Pathology
- 4.9 Theme: Dental Caries
- 4.10 Theme: Dental Caries – Epidemiology
- 4.11 Theme: Dental Caries – Histology
- 4.12 Theme: Ameloblastoma
- 4.13 Theme: Osteosarcoma
- 4.14 Theme: Radicular Cysts (1)
- 4.15 Theme: Radicular Cysts (2)
- 4.16 Theme: Dentigerous Cysts (1)
- 4.17 Theme: Dentigerous Cysts (2)
- 4.18 Theme: Odontogenic Keratocysts – Epidemiology
- 4.19 Theme: Odontogenic Keratocysts
- 4.20 Theme: Other Cysts
- 4.21 Theme: Odontogenic Tumours
- 4.22 Theme: Multiple Myeloma
- 4.23 Theme: Syphilis
- 4.24 Theme: Fibrous Dysplasia
- 4.25 Theme: Paget's Disease
- 4.26 Theme: Kaposi's Sarcoma

4.1 Theme: Autoantibodies/Autoimmune Diseases

A   Addison's disease
B   Goodpasture syndrome
C   Graves' disease
D   Guillain–Barré syndrome
E   Type 1 diabetes
F   Lambert–Eaton myasthenic syndrome
G   Myasthenia gravis
H   Primary biliary cirrhosis

From the options listed above which diseases do antibodies to the following antigens cause? You may use each option once, more than once or not at all.

1   Acetylcholine receptor
2   Glutamic acid decarboxylase
3   Beta cells in islets of Langerhans
4   Mitochondria
5   Peripheral nerve myelin component
6   Thyroid stimulating hormone receptor

4.2 Theme: Cranial Nerves

A   Olfactory nerve (Cranial nerve I)
B   Optic nerve (Cranial nerve II)
C   Oculomotor nerve (Cranial nerve III)
D   Trochlear nerve (Cranial nerve IV)
E   Trigeminal nerve (Cranial nerve V)
F   Abducens nerve (Cranial nerve VI)
G   Facial nerve (Cranial nerve VII)
H   Vestibulocochlear nerve (Cranial nerve VIII)
I   Glossopharyngeal nerve (Cranial nerve IX)
J   Vagus nerve (Cranial nerve X)
K   Accessory nerve (Cranial nerve XI)
L   Hypoglossal nerve (Cranial nerve XII)

For each of the following clinical scenarios, choose the affected cranial nerve from the list above. You may use each option once, more than once or not at all.

1   A 32 year-old woman woke up to find the right side of her face drooping. She had difficulty blinking with the right eyelid and found food tasted funny.

2   A man is having difficulty swallowing. When he says 'aah' the uvula moves across to the right. The vagus nerve is clearly affected, which other nerve is involved?

3   A patient is experiencing double vision. This occurs when she looks towards the right. When she attempts to do this, his right eye fails to abduct. Which nerve is affected in the right eye?

4   A 45 year-old patient complains of persistent anaesthesia affecting the lower lip after a recent third molar extraction.

5   A man complains double vision in most directions of gaze. He has an obvious ptosis of the left eye. When the eyelid is pulled up, the left eye is observed to be depressed and out towards the lateral canthus of the eye.

4.3 Theme: Peripheral Nerve Injuries

A Cervical sympathetic chain
B Facial nerve
C Hypoglossal nerve
D Long thoracic nerve of Bell
E Nerve roots C5 and C6
F Trigeminal nerve
G Radial nerve
H Ulnar nerve

For the following statements, choose the most closely associated cranial nerve from the list above. You may use each option once, more than once or not at all.

1 Bell's palsy.
2 Injury results in Erb's palsy.
3 Injury causes paralysis of serratus anterior muscle.
4 Horner syndrome.
5 Miosis, ptosis, vasodilatation and anhidrosis of the face.

4.4 Theme: Skin Infections

A *Candida albicans*
B Herpes simplex virus
C Human papilloma virus
D Impetigo
E *Molluscum contagiosum*
F *Prevotella intermedia*
G Varicella zoster virus

For the following conditions, choose the most appropriate causative organism from the list above. You may use each option once, more than once or not at all.

1 Crusted lesions on the lip.
2 Viral warts.
3 Cutaneous infection of childhood caused by a pox virus.
4 Highly infectious, spread by direct contact, presenting as honey crusted lesions.
5 Shingles.

4.5 Theme: Systemic Conditions Associated with Root Resorption

A	Gaucher's disease
B	Goltz syndrome
C	Hyperparathyroidism
D	Hypoparathyroidism
E	Hypophosphataemia
F	Hyperphosphataemia
G	Paget's disease of bone
H	Papillon–Lefèvre syndrome
I	Turner syndrome

For each of the statements below, choose the option more closely associated with root resorption from the list above. You may use each option once, more than once or not at all.

1. Congenital condition causing palmoplantar hyperkeratosis and juvenile periodontitis.
2. Bone disease characterised by total disorganization of bone remodelling.
3. Affects females only who have short stature, low hairline and web neck with a complete or partial deletion of chromosome X.
4. X-linked disorder with multiple mesenchymal defects, skin lesions, oral warts and dental defects.
5. Deficiency of the enzyme glucocerebrosidase and lipid storage disorder. May cause dry mouth and is the most common genetic disease affecting Ashkenazi Jewish people of Eastern European ancestry.

4.6 Theme: Eponymous Syndromes

A	Apert syndrome	E	Marfan syndrome
B	Ehlers–Danlos syndrome	F	Papillion-Lefèvre syndrome
C	Heerfordt syndrome	G	Ramsey-Hunt syndrome
D	Larsen syndrome	H	Stickler syndrome

For each of the following scenarios, select the most appropriate option from the list above. You may use each option once, more than once or not at all.

1. A syndrome comprising hyperflexibility of joints, increased bleeding and hyperextensible skin. The abnormality is an underlying collagen defect.

2. A syndrome of sarcoidosis with lacrimal and salivary gland swelling (usually parotid), uveitis and fever. Occasionally, there are neuropathies such as facial nerve palsy.

3. A syndrome of palm and sole hyperkeratosis and juvenile periodontitis affecting the primary and secondary dentition.

4.7 Theme: Oral 'Lumps and Bumps'

A	Acute oral thrush
B	Developmental periodontal cysts
C	Epstein's pearls
D	Eruption cyst
E	Fordyce's spots
F	Kaposi's sarcoma
G	Mucocele
H	Mucoepidermoid carcinoma
I	Oral keratosis

For each of the following scenarios, select the most appropriate option from the list above. You may use each option once, more than once or not at all.

1. A 16-year-old boy presents with a 1 cm bluish lesion on his lower lip. The lesion is painless with no discharge but the boy feels it may be getting bigger.

2. A 65-year-old non-smoker is referred to the oral surgery department with multiple bilateral, 'pin-head' sized, buccal lesions, which are cream-coloured and well demarcated. They are painless and have been present for a long time.

3. A 1-month-old child is referred by his paediatrician with lumpy gums. A number of small cysts are seen on the alveolar ridge, which resolve by age 4 months.

4.8 Theme: Oropharyngeal Pathology

A Basal cell carcinoma
B Candidiasis
C Crohn's disease
D Kaposi's sarcoma
E Local infection
F Oral hairy leukoplakia
G Squamous cell carcinoma
H Tetracycline
I Ulcerative colitis
J Vitamin C deficiency

For each of the following statements, choose the most appropriate diagnosis from the list above. You may use each option once, more than once or not at all.

1 A 24-year-old man presents complaining of recurrent mouth ulcers and recent change in bowel habit.

2 An 81-year-old female patient with a history of chronic obstructive pulmonary disease, who is on repeat prescription for steroid inhalers.

3 A 72-year-old man who is smoker and is complaining of a solitary yet persistent ulcer on the side of his tongue.

4 A 42-year-old newly diagnosed human immunodeficiency virus (HIV)- positive patient presents with painless white plaques on his tongue.

5 A 41-year-old African immigrant presents with a reddish-brown papule on his hard palate.

ORAL PATHOLOGY

4.9 Theme: Dental Caries

A	Clarke
B	Jones
C	Miller
D	Acid-chelation
E	Acidogenic
F	Proteolytic
G	1
H	2
I	3
J	4
K	5
L	*Actinomyces*
M	*Lactobacillus*
N	*Prevotella intermedia*
O	*Streptococcus milleri*
P	*Streptococcus mutans*

'The acid formed from the fermentation of dietary carbohydrates by oral bacteria leads to the progressive demineralisation of tooth substance with subsequent disintegration of the organic matrix'.

For each of the following questions about the statement above, choose the most appropriate option from the list. You may use each option once, more than once or not at all.

1. Whose theory is this?
2. What is the theory called?
3. How many elements are there to this theory?
4. Which bacterium is most commonly found in enamel caries?
5. Which bacterium is most commonly found in root caries?
6. Which bacterium is most commonly found at the advancing edge of caries?

4.10 Theme: Dental Caries – Epidemiology

A   Vipeholm
B   Niilstrom
C   Hopewood House
D   Easter Island
E   Tristan da Cunha
F   Christmas Island
G   Turku–xylitol
H   Gnotobiotic mice
I   Gnotobiotic rats
J   Istanbul – sucrose substitute
K   Hurler syndrome
L   Hunter syndrome
M   Hereditary fructose intolerance

For each of the following descriptions of epidemiological studies, choose the most appropriate name from the list above. You may use each option once, more than once or not at all.

1. An Australian children's home where the diet was extremely regimented. The children were denied sweets and white bread. During their stay in the home, various children's caries incidence was very low, but after they left, their caries incidence increased.

2. A study on a hereditary condition in which children physically are unable to tolerate one of the causes of caries. In people affected by this condition the incidence of caries is low.

3. A study on a small island in the Pacific that had low dental caries incidence prior to the arrival of American troops in the Second World War. After the Americans arrived with sweets and carbonated drinks, the caries incidence rose dramatically.

4. A study which showed a 90% decrease in dental caries in children, when sugar was substituted by an alternative sweetener.

5. A study conducted at a home for people with learning difficulties, where patients were split into various groups. Some were only given sticky toffee at mealtimes, while others were given sticky toffee on demand. There was a large difference in the prevalence of caries in each group.

6. Certain animals were kept germ-free and given the same diet as other animals which were non-germ-free. The germ-free animals did not get dental caries, whereas the non-germ-free animals did get caries.

4.11 Theme: Dental Caries – Histology

A	Body of lesion
B	Dark zone
C	Surface zone
D	Translucent zone
E	Zone of bacterial invasion
F	Zone of demineralisation
G	Zone of destruction
H	Zone of sclerosis

For each of the following statements, choose the most appropriate option from the list above. You may use each option once, more than once or not at all.

1. The histopathological zone closest to the advancing edge of enamel caries.
2. The histopathological zone second closest to the advancing edge of enamel caries.
3. The histopathological zone third closest to the advancing edge of enamel caries.
4. The histopathological zone outermost to the advancing edge of enamel caries.
5. The histopathological zone closest to the advancing edge of dentinal caries.
6. The histopathological zone second closest to the advancing edge of dentinal caries.
7. The histopathological zone third closest to the advancing edge of dentinal caries.
8. The histopathological zone outermost to the advancing edge of dentinal caries.

4.12 Theme: Ameloblastoma

A	Male
B	Female
C	Equally prevalent in males and females
D	0–18 years
E	18–25 years
F	25–40 years
G	40+ years
H	Anterior maxilla
I	Posterior maxilla
J	Anterior mandible
K	Posterior mandible
L	Basal cell type
M	Follicular
N	Granular
O	Plexiform
P	Single
Q	Multilocular
R	Multiple
S	Metastasises
T	Does not metastasise

For each of the following questions, choose the most appropriate option from the list above. You may use each option once, more than once or not at all.

1. Which sex does ameloblastoma mainly occur in?
2. Which age group does it most commonly occur in?
3. Where is it usually found?
4. What is the most common type of ameloblastoma?
5. Is it single, multilocular or multiple?
6. Does it metastasise?

4.13 Theme: Osteosarcoma

A Male
B Female
C Equally prevalent in males and females
D Under 18 years
E 18–30 years
F 30–50 years
G 50+ years
H Fibroblasts
I Osteoblasts
J Osteoclasts
K Mandible
L Maxilla
M Frontal
N Temporal
O Brain
P Kidneys
Q Liver
R Lungs
S 20%
T 40%
U 60%
V 80%

For each of the following questions, choose the most appropriate option from the list above. You may use each option once, more than once or not at all.

1 Which sex does osteosarcoma mostly occur in?
2 Which age group does it mostly affect?
3 Which cells are most commonly abnormal?
4 Which bone in the skull is most commonly affected?
5 Where does it metastasise to?
6 What is the 5-year survival prognosis?

4.14 Theme: Radicular Cysts (1)

A	Male
B	Female
C	Under 18 years
D	18–30 years
E	30–50 years
F	50+ years
G	Incidental finding
H	Mobility of associated tooth
I	Obvious swelling
J	Pain associated with the tooth
K	Mandibular wisdom teeth
L	Maxillary wisdom teeth
M	Maxillary incisors
N	Mandibular incisors
O	Developmental
P	Congenital
Q	Trauma
R	Vital
S	Non-vital

For each of the following questions, choose the most appropriate option from the list above. You may use each option once, more than once or not at all.

1 In which sex are radicular cysts most prevalent?
2 In which age group do they most commonly occur?
3 How are they commonly discovered?
4 Which teeth do they most commonly affect?
5 What is the most common cause?
6 What is the status of the pulp in this condition?

ORAL PATHOLOGY

4.15 Theme: Radicular Cysts (2)

A	Root sheath of Hertwig
B	Rests of Malassez
C	Reduced enamel epithelium
D	Glands of Serres
E	Enamel organ
F	10%
G	25%
H	50%
I	75%
J	Cuboidal
K	Stratified squamous
L	Columnar
M	Cholesterol
N	Calcium
O	Fat
P	Nothing, it will spontaneously heal
Q	Extraction of affected tooth
R	Enucleation

For each of the following questions, choose the most appropriate option from the list above. You may use each option once, more than once or not at all.

1. Which epithelial residue proliferates to form radicular cysts?
2. What is this epithelial residue derived from?
3. What proportion of all jaw cysts are radicular cysts?
4. Which epithelium makes up the cyst lining?
5. What chemical is frequently found in these cysts?
6. What is the appropriate treatment?

4.16 Theme: Dentigerous Cysts (1)

A   Male
B   Female
C   Equally prevalent among males and females
D   Under 18 years
E   18–30 years
F   30–50 years
G   50+ years
H   Maxillary wisdom teeth
I   Mandibular wisdom teeth
J   Maxillary canines
K   Mandibular premolars
L   Root sheath of Hertwig
M   Rests of Malassez
N   Glands of Serres
O   Reduced enamel epithelium
P   Enamel organ

For each of the following questions, choose the most appropriate option from the list above. You may use each option once, more than once or not at all.

1. Which sex is most commonly affected?
2. In which age group is a dentigerous cyst first noticed?
3. Which teeth are most commonly affected?
4. Which teeth are second-most-commonly affected?
5. Which epithelial residue is responsible for the formation of this cyst?
6. From what is the epithelial tissue in Q 5 derived?

ORAL PATHOLOGY

4.17 Theme: Dentigerous Cysts (2)

A	Developmental
B	Inflammatory
C	0–5%
D	5–10%
E	10–15%
F	15–20%
G	Epidermal cyst
H	Eruption cyst
I	Gingival cyst
J	Columnar
K	Cuboidal
L	Stratified squamous
M	None of it, it is separate
N	The crown
O	The root
P	The whole tooth
Q	Enucleation
R	Excision and extraction of the tooth
S	Nothing, it will resolve spontaneously

For each of the following questions, choose the most appropriate option from the list above. You may use each option once, more than once or not at all.

1. Are these developmental or inflammatory cysts?
2. What proportion of all dental cysts do dentigerous cysts make up?
3. If a dentigerous cyst is found in the overlying gingivae, what is it called?
4. What cells make up the lining of the cyst?
5. Which part of the tooth does a dentigerous cyst encompass?
6. What is the treatment for a dentigerous cyst?

4.18 Theme: Odontogenic Keratocysts – Epidemiology

A	Male
B	Female
C	Equally prevalent in males and females
D	0–16 years
E	16–30 years
F	30–40 years
G	40–50 years
H	50–70 years
I	1%
J	5%
K	10%
L	15%
M	20%
N	Rests of Malassez
O	Root sheath of Hertwig
P	Reduced enamel epithelium
Q	Enamel organ
R	Glands of Serres

For each of the following questions, choose the most appropriate option from the list above. You may use each option once, more than once or not at all.

1. In which sex are odontogenic keratocysts more common?
2. In which age group is there the earliest peak of incidence?
3. In which other age group is there also a peak of incidence?
4. What proportion of odontogenic cysts do these cysts form?
5. From which developmental residue do odontogenic keratocysts arise?

4.19 Theme: Odontogenic Keratocysts

A   Maxillary posterior region
B   Mandibular posterior region
C   Maxillary anterior region
D   Mandibular anterior region
E   Columnar
F   Cuboidal
G   Stratified squamous keratinising epithelium
H   Stratified squamous non-keratinising epithelium
I   1–2 cells
J   5–8 cells
K   15–30 cells
L   30+ cells
M   Enucleation
N   Enucleation with curettage
O   Nothing, it will spontaneously resolve
P   Hyperkeratinised
Q   Orthokeratinised
R   Parakeratinised
S   Down syndrome
T   Gorlin–Goltz syndrome
U   Larsen syndrome

For each of the following questions, choose the most appropriate option from the list above. You may use each option once, more than once or not at all.

1. Where are odontogenic keratocysts most commonly found?
2. Which type of cell forms the cyst lining?
3. How many cells thick is the cyst lining?
4. What is the treatment of choice?
5. Which type of odontogenic keratocyst tends to recur?
6. Which syndrome is associated with multiple odontogenic keratocysts?

4.20 Theme: Other Cysts

- A   Aneurysmal bone cyst
- B   Calcifying odontogenic cyst
- C   Globulomaxillary cyst
- D   Nasolabial cyst
- E   Nasopalatine cyst
- F   Solitary bone cyst

For each of the following descriptions, choose the most appropriate diagnosis from the list above. You may use each option once, more than once or not at all.

1. A midline cyst of the anterior maxilla with lining of squamous and/or ciliated columnar epithelium. Characteristically there may be a neurovascular bundle and sometimes salivary acini found in the cyst wall.

2. A developmental cyst which forms in the anterior maxilla between the lateral incisor and canine. Both of these teeth are vital. The cyst has a fibrous wall which may be squamous columnar or columnar ciliated.

3. This is a rare soft tissue cyst external to the alveolar ridge below the ala nasi. It probably arises from the remnants of the lower end of the nasolacrimal duct. Peak incidence is 40–50 years.

4. Although cystic, this lesion can be solid and may be a benign odontogenic tumour. Most commonly occurs in the second decade. It has a fibrous wall with a lining of squamous epithelium, but the basal layer may be columnar and ameloblast-like. Abnormal keratinisation of spinous cells produces 'ghost cells'. There is patchy calcification.

5. This is possibly a developmental defect or result of bleeding into, or vascularisation of, a pre-existing lesion such as a giant cell granuloma.

6. Almost invariably occurs in the mandible. The cavity and radiolucency extend through cancellous bone and arch up between the roots of teeth but rarely expand the bone. The cyst cavity may contain serosanguineous fluid or may be empty. This cyst is unusual in that it may heal spontaneously.

4.21 Theme: Odontogenic Tumours

A	Ameloblastic fibroma
B	Ameloblastoma
C	Calcifying epithelial odontogenic tumour
D	Cementoma
E	Complex odontome
F	Compound odontome
G	Odontogenic myxoma
H	Squamous odontogenic tumour

For each of the following descriptions, choose the most appropriate option from the list above. You may use each option once, more than once or not at all.

1. Multiple small tooth-like structures (denticles) found within follicles.

2. A rare tumour that typically affects teenagers. There is a slow-growing painless swelling with a cyst-like area of radiolucency. A biopsy shows processes of epithelium resembling stellate reticulum. The stroma represents dentine. This is thought to be a true mixed tumour and is sometimes associated with a composite developing odontome.

3. A completely irregular mass of dental tissues. It may have a cauliflower form with dental tissues surrounding a much branched pulp chamber. Although it lacks any morphological resemblance to a tooth, this lesion has individual dental tissues in normal relation to one another.

4. A rare but important tumour because of its resemblance, and risk of confusion with a poorly differentiated carcinoma. The radiographic appearance is variable, but is classically described as diffuse radiolucency often with scattered snow-shower opacities.

5. The most common neoplasm of the jaws. It chiefly affects males over the age of 40 years, and occurs mainly in the posterior body or ramus of the mandible. There are several types, including follicular, plexiform, acanthomatous and basal. It may recur, and requires excision with a 2 cm margin.

6. This tumour usually affects males under 25 years of age. It appears as a radiopaque apical mass, well attached to a tooth with radiolucent margin, usually in the molar region. It is probably a benign tumour.

4.22 Theme: Multiple Myeloma

A 0–18 years
B 18–35 years
C 35–60 years
D 60+ years
E Male
F Female
G Equally prevalent in males and females
H African-Caribbean
I Asian
J Caucasian
K Electric shock appearance
L Hyperdense bony appearance
M Pepper pot skull
N Epithelial
O Osteoblast
P Plasma
Q Bence Jones
R Graham
S Williams

For each of the following questions, choose the most appropriate option from the list above. You may use each option once, more than once or not at all.

1 What is the most common age group of presentation for multiple myeloma?
2 In which sex is it more prevalent?
3 In which ethnic group is it most prevalent?
4 What is the classic finding on a skull X-ray?
5 Multiple myeloma is a tumour of which cell?
6 Which protein in the urine is diagnostic for this condition?

4.23 Theme: Syphilis

A Chlamydia trichomatosis
B Clostridium botulinum
C Treponema pallidum
D Albright
E Hutchinson
F Markowitz
G Mulberry
H Jones
I Chancre
J Snail track
K Tabes dorsalis
L Gumma
M Aortic aneurysm
N Mitral stenosis
O Pulmonary coarctation

For each of the following questions, choose the most appropriate option from the list above. You may use each option once, more than once or not at all.

1 What is the causative organism of syphilis called?
2 In congenital syphilis, what is the name of the deformed incisors associated with this condition?
3 In congenital syphilis, what is the name of the deformed molars associated with this condition?
4 In secondary syphilis, what is the name of the ulcers found in the mouth?
5 What is the name of the intra-oral lesions in the mouth which are found in tertiary syphilis?
6 Which cardiovascular complication is associated with tertiary syphilis?

ORAL PATHOLOGY 157

4.24 Theme: Fibrous Dysplasia

A	Male
B	Female
C	Equally prevalent in males and females
D	0–16 years
E	16–30 years
F	30–50 years
G	50+ years
H	Frontal bone
I	Temporal bone
J	Maxilla
K	Mandible
L	Ground glass
M	Radio-opacity
N	Snow storm
O	Disfigurement and malocclusion
P	Nothing, incidental finding
Q	Pain
R	No treatment, spontaneous arrest of progress with skeletal maturity
S	Urgent resection due to malignant potential

For each of the following questions, choose the most appropriate option from the list above. You may use each option once, more than once or not at all.

1 In which sex is this condition most prevalent?
2 In which age group is the condition most commonly found?
3 Where in the head is this condition most commonly found?
4 What is the classic radiographic appearance?
5 What do patients usually complain of at initial presentation?
6 What is the treatment in most patients?

ORAL PATHOLOGY

4.25 Theme: Paget's Disease

A	18-30 years
B	30-50 years
C	50+ years
D	0.5%
E	1%
F	5%
G	15%
H	Feet
I	Maxilla
J	Pelvis
K	Ribs
L	Alkaline phosphatase
M	Calcium
N	Haemoglobin
O	Analgesics
P	Antibiotics
Q	Steroids
R	Life-long
S	1 year
T	5 years
U	10 years

For each of the following questions, choose the most appropriate option from the list above. You may use each option once, more than once or not at all.

1. In which age group does Paget's disease present?
2. In what percentage of the population is it radiologically detectable?
3. Which bone does it affect most commonly?
4. Which biological marker aids diagnosis?
5. What should you prescribe to Paget's patients after a routine extraction?
6. How long is the disease active for?

4.26 Theme: Kaposi's Sarcoma

A Male
B Female
C Equally prevalent in males and females
D HIV
E Human papilloma virus
F Paramyxovirus
G Human herpesvirus
H Red
I Yellow
J Pink
K Purple
L Epithelial
M Endothelial
N Bone
O Muscle
P 6 months
Q 1 year
R 2 years
S 5 years
T Life-long, it is benign

For each of the following questions, choose the most appropriate option from the list above. You may use each option once, more than once or not at all.

1. In which sex is Kaposi's sarcoma most prevalent?
2. Which virus is the causative organism for this condition?
3. Which virus is the virus in Q 2 associated with?
4. What colour is the lesion in the mouth?
5. Which tissue is this a tumour of?
6. What is the mean survival time from diagnosis to death?

ORAL PATHOLOGY

4.1 Autoantibodies/Autoimmune Diseases

1 G Myasthenia gravis

2 E Type 1 diabetes

3 E Type 1 diabetes

4 H Primary biliary cirrhosis

5 D Guillain-Barré Syndrome

6 C Graves' disease

Autoimmune diseases arise from an abnormal immune response of the body against substances and tissues normally present in the body (autoimmunity).

Myasthenia gravis is a neuromuscular disease that leads to fluctuating muscle weakness and fatigue. In the most common cases, muscle weakness is caused by circulating antibodies that block acetylcholine receptors at the postsynaptic neuromuscular junction.

Type 1 diabetes (formerly insulin-dependent diabetes or juvenile diabetes) is a form of diabetes mellitus that results from the autoimmune destruction of the insulin-producing beta cells (cells in the islets of Langerhans) in the pancreas. Both glutamic acid decarboxylase GAD_{67} and GAD_{65} are targets of autoantibodies in people who later develop type 1 diabetes mellitus or latent autoimmune diabetes. Injections with GAD_{65} have been shown to preserve some insulin production for 30 months in humans with type 1 diabetes.

Primary biliary cirrhosis (PBC) is an autoimmune disease of the liver. Cirrhosis is only a feature of advanced disease, and a change of name has been proposed. Most of the patients (>90%) have anti-mitochondrial antibodies (AMAs).

Guillain-Barré syndrome (GBS), also known as Guillain-Barré–Strohl syndrome or Landry's paralysis, is a rapid-onset muscle weakness as a result of damage to the peripheral nervous system. Two-thirds of people with Guillain-Barré syndrome have experienced an infection before the onset of the condition. The nerve dysfunction in Guillain-Barré syndrome is caused by an immune attack on the nerve cells of the peripheral nervous system and their support structures.

Graves' disease, also known as toxic diffuse goiter, is an autoimmune disease that affects the thyroid. Autoantibodies bind to the thyroid stimulating hormone receptor resulting in high levels of circulating thyroid hormones.

4.2 Cranial Nerves

| 1 | G | Facial nerve |

| 2 | I | Glossopharyngeal nerve |

| 3 | F | Abducens nerve |

| 4 | E | Trigeminal nerve |

| 5 | C | Oculomotor |

The patient in Q1 has a Bell's palsy, ie a lower motor neurone lesion of the facial nerve. It is a lower motor neurone lesion because of the inability to close the eyelid on the affected side. Because taste is affected, the chorda tympani branch of the facial nerve must also be affected.

The uvula moves away from the affected side, so it will be the left vagus and glossopharyngeal muscles that are affected.

The patient in Q3 should have a convergent squint as well.

The inferior alveolar nerve (inferior dental nerve) is a branch of the mandibular nerve of the third division of the trigeminal. This nerve supplies sensation to the lower lip and may be damaged if the roots of the third molar are in close anatomical relations to the nerve when an extraction is done.

The eye's position of being 'down and out' gives a big clue to a third-nerve palsy. Ptosis is also another feature, and it pays to lift up the eyelid to examine the eye beneath so this (and other pathology) is not missed.

ORAL PATHOLOGY

4.3 Peripheral Nerve Injuries

1	B	Facial nerve
2	E	Nerve roots C5 and C6
3	D	Long thoracic nerve of Bell
4	A	Cervical sympathetic chain
5	A	Cervical sympathetic chain

Bell's palsy is caused by damage to the facial nerve, which supplies motor innervation to the facial muscles. Most likely this results from compression of the facial nerve within its canal, usually owing to infection. Viral infection is common and causes swelling and inflammation of the nerve.

Erb's palsy (also known as Erb–Duchenne palsy) is a paralysis of the arm caused by injury to the upper group of the arm's main nerves, specifically the severing of the upper trunk C5–C6 nerves.

The long thoracic nerve (external respiratory nerve of Bell; posterior thoracic nerve) supplies the serratus anterior muscle.

Horner syndrome (occulosympathetic palsy) is a combination of symptoms that arises when a group of nerves known as the sympathetic trunk is damaged. It is characterised by unilateral miosis (a constricted pupil), partial ptosis (a weak, droopy eyelid), and apparent anhidrosis (loss of sweating on the same side, depending upon the extent of the lesion), with or without enophthalmus (inset eyeball). Hence Q 5 is a description of Horner syndrome.

4.4 Skin Infections

1 B Herpes simplex virus

2 C Human papilloma virus

3 E *Molluscum contagiosum*

4 D Impetigo

5 G Varicella zoster virus

Herpes labialis (also called cold sores, fever blisters, herpes simplex labialis, recurrent herpes labialis, or orolabial herpes) is a type of herpes simplex occurring on the lip, i.e. an infection caused by herpes simplex virus (HSV). The latent virus can be reactivated in patients, often up to 30% presenting with 'cold sores'. It can be triggered by febrile conditions, common cold, menstruation, exposure to strong sunshine and other insults.

Human papilloma virus establishes productive infections only in keratinocytes of the skin or mucous membranes, and these benign papillomas may become warts or squamous cell papillomas.

Molluscum contagiosum is a viral infection of the skin or occasionally of the mucous membranes, sometimes called water warts. The virus that causes the infection is spread from person to person by touching the affected skin.

Impetigo is a highly contagious bacterial skin infection most common among preschool children.

Shingles, also known as zoster, herpes zoster, or zona, is a viral disease characterised by a painful skin rash with blisters involving a limited area. Shingles is due to a reactivation of varicella zoster virus (VZV) after a previous initial infection which causes chicken pox.

Candida albicans causes fungal infections and *Prevotella intermedia* is associated with periodontal disease.

4.5 Systemic Conditions Associated with Root Resorption

1 H Papillon–Lefèvre syndrome

2 G Paget's disease of bone

3 I Turner syndrome

4 B Goltz syndrome

5 A Gaucher's disease

Hyperparathyroidism is usually due to a parathyroid adenoma or hyperplasia of the parathyroid tissue. Oral manifestations are reduced bone density with less distinct outlines of the maxillary sinus and ID canals on a radiograph as well as root resorption. Systemic manifestations include renal stones, bone lesions, polyuria and abdominal pain.

Hypoparathyroidism is usually caused by damage to the parathyroid tissue. Clinical manifestations are associated with low calcium levels. Oral paresthesia and facial nerve stimulation may result in involuntary facial muscle twitching.

Hypophosphataemia is an electrolyte disturbance with low phosphate levels in the blood and is the most common cause of non-nutritional rickets.

Hyperphosphataemia is an electrolyte disturbance with elevated phosphate levels in the blood that can result in chronic renal failure.

4.6 Eponymous Syndromes

1 B Ehlers–Danlos syndrome (EDS)

EDS encompasses several types of inherited connective tissue disorders. Connective tissue provides support to parts of the body such as the skin and muscles, but in EDS the collagen that gives strength and elasticity to connective tissue is faulty. This results in hyperelastic skin that is fragile and bruises easily, excessive looseness of the joints, blood vessels that are easily damaged and, rarely, rupture of internal organs.

2 C Heerfordt syndrome

This is an acute syndromal presentation of sarcoidosis, and has the following features:

- Fever
- Uveitis
- Swelling of parotid ± other salivary/lacrimal glands.

3 F Papillon–Lefèvre syndrome

Papillon–Lefèvre syndrome is a rare autosomal recessive disorder characterised by hyperkeratosis of the palms and soles and severe destructive periodontal disease, affecting both the primary and permanent teeth.

4.7 Oral 'Lumps and Bumps'

1 G Mucocele

This is the classic presentation of a mucocele and can be removed by surgery or cryotherapy.

2 E Fordyce's spots

Lesions which have been present for years and are small, well demarcated and painless would lead to the conclusion of Fordyce spots; these are sebaceous glands.

3 C Epstein's pearls

This is the classic description of gingival cysts (Epstein's pearls and Bohn's nodules), which arise from remnants of the dental lamina that proliferates to form a keratinising (white) cyst; they are often multiple.

4.8 Oropharyngeal Pathology

1 C Crohn's disease

Crohn's disease is a subdivision of inflammatory bowel disease. In Crohn's any part of the gastrointestinal tract from the mouth to the anus may be affected. Recurrent aphthous ulcers, abdominal pain, diarrhoea ± blood and weight loss are common symptoms.

2 B Candidiasis

Recurrent steroid inhaler use (if spacer devices are not used) predisposes to oral candidiasis secondary to immunosuppression.

3 G Squamous cell carcinoma

Squamous cell carcinoma of the oropharynx may present as a poorly healing mouth ulcer that may bleed intermittently, have hard, raised edges and an irregular border. Smoking is a recognised risk factor.

4 F Oral hairy leukoplakia

Clinically, oral hairy leukoplakia appears as white patch(es) on the lateral border of the tongue and is caused by the Epstein–Barr virus. This manifestation is consistent with severe defects of immunity such as HIV infection.

5 D Kaposi's sarcoma

Oral Kaposi's sarcoma predominately presents as red-brown nodules on the hard palate or gums. This disease is caused by human herpesvirus 8 (HHV-8) and is consistently found in immunocompromised patients such as those with AIDS or on immunosuppressants following organ transplantation.

ORAL PATHOLOGY

4.9 Dental Caries

1	C	Miller
2	E	Acidogenic
3	J	4
4	P	*Streptococcus mutans*
5	L	*Actinomyces*
6	M	*Lactobacillus*

Miller in 1889 proposed the acidogenic theory, in which he described four elements required to produce dental caries – tooth substance, bacteria, substrate and, crucially, time.

4.10 Dental Caries – Epidemiology

1	C	Hopewood House
2	M	Hereditary fructose intolerance
3	E	Tristan da Cunha
4	G	Turku-xylitol
5	A	Vipeholm
6	I	Gnotobiotic rats

4.11 Dental Caries – Histology

1 D Translucent zone

2 B Dark zone

3 A Body of lesion

4 C Surface zone

5 H Zone of sclerosis

6 F Zone of demineralisation

7 E Zone of bacterial invasion

8 G Zone of destruction

The four zones of enamel caries in order from the advancing edge	The four zones of dentinal caries in order from the advancing edge
1. Translucent zone	1. Zone of sclerosis
2. Dark zone	2. Zone of demineralisation
3. Body of lesion	3. Zone of bacterial invasion
4. Surface zone	4. Zone of destruction

4.12 Ameloblastoma

1 A Male

2 G 40+ years

3 K Posterior mandible

4 M Follicular

5 Q Multilocular

6 T Does not metastasise

Ameloblastoma is the most common neoplasm of the jaws. It mainly affects males over the age of 40 years, with about 80% of the tumours occurring in the ramus or posterior body of the mandible. It typically appears as a multilocular cyst: rarely is it monolocular, and it never occurs at multiple different sites. It is slow-growing and locally invasive but does not metastasise. Treatment is by complete excision with a 2 cm margin of normal bone. However, it does tend to recur, and regular follow-up is needed.

4.13 Osteosarcoma

1 A Male

2 D Under 18 years

3 I Osteoblasts

4 K Mandible

5 R Lungs

6 T 40%

Osteosarcoma is the most common primary bone tumour. It can be a rare complication of Paget's disease or occur as a result of radiotherapy. It mostly affects young males. The tumour consists of abnormal tumour osteoblasts, which are typically angular, hyperchromatic and larger than normal. Surrounding bone is usually destroyed. Clinically, there is a rapidly growing soft tissue mass with a ragged area of radiolucency and radiopacity with no definable pattern. Metastasis occurs to the lung with typical cannon ball radiopacities. The 5-year survival is 40%.

4.14 Radicular Cysts (1)

1 A Male

2 E 30–50 years

3 G Incidental finding

4 M Maxillary incisors

5 Q Trauma

6 S Non-vital

Radicular cysts are commonly found as an incidental finding in a patient's fourth or fifth decade. The most common cause is trauma, which accounts for the greater prevalence being in the male population. Associated teeth are non-vital. Although all the options with regard to presentation are possible, incidental finding is the most common presentation.

4.15 Radicular Cysts (2)

1 B Rests of Malassez

2 A Root sheath of Hertwig

3 I 75%

4 K Stratified squamous

5 M Cholesterol

6 R Enucleation

The lining of radicular cysts consists of stratified squamous epithelium. The entire lining is variable in thickness; sometimes with arcaded configuration, irregularly acanthotic or occasionally very thick. In most cases the thick epithelial wall allows the enucleation of the cyst from its bony wall. Aetiology of these cysts may be: pulp death; apical periodontitis; proliferation of the epithelial rests of Malassez; cystic change in the epithelium; expansion of the cyst by hydrostatic pressure; resorption of bone. This is an inflammatory cyst.

4.16 Dentigerous Cysts (1)

1 A Male

2 E 18–30 years

3 I Mandibular wisdom teeth

4 K Mandibular premolars

5 O Reduced enamel epithelium

6 P Enamel organ

4.17 Dentigerous Cysts (2)

1	A	Developmental
2	F	15-20%
3	H	Eruption cyst
4	L	Stratified squamous
5	N	The crown
6	R	Excision and extraction of the tooth

The pathogenesis of a dentigerous cyst involves the cystic change of the enamel organ after the completion of enamel formation. This is a developmental defect of unknown cause. These cysts are twice as common in men as in women. The cyst wall is attached to the neck of the tooth at the amelocemental junction. The lining of the cyst is a thin, flat layer of squamous cells without a defined basal layer. An eruption cyst is strictly a soft tissue cyst in the gingivae overlying an unerupted tooth.

4.18 Odontogenic Keratocysts – Epidemiology

1	A	Male
2	E	16-30 years
3	G	40-50 years
4	K	10%
5	R	Glands of Serres

4.19 Odontogenic Keratocysts

1 B Mandibular posterior region

2 G Stratified squamous keratinising epithelium

3 J 5-8 cells

4 N Enucleation with curettage

5 R Parakeratinised

6 T Gorlin-Goltz

Odontogenic keratocysts arise in the posterior mandible, mainly the body and ramus. A tooth is sometimes missing. They comprise 10% of all odontogenic cysts, and the male to female ratio is 1.5:1. They form most frequently in young adults and in people between 50 and 60 years of age. There is a characteristic lining of epithelium of even thickness, 5-8 cells thick, with a flat basement membrane. There is a layer of tall palisaded basal cells and a thin eosinophilic layer of parakeratin.

4.20 Other Cysts

1 E Nasopalatine cyst

2 C Globulomaxillary cyst

3 D Nasolabial cyst

4 B Calcifying odontogenic cyst

5 A Aneurysmal bone cyst

6 F Solitary bone cyst

Non-odontogenic cysts should not be forgotten, as they can be asked about. But if you are short of time for revision, revise the odontogenic cysts first.

ORAL PATHOLOGY

4.21 Odontogenic Tumours

1	F	Compound odontome
2	A	Ameloblastic fibroma
3	E	Complex odontome
4	C	Calcifying epithelial odontogenic tumour
5	B	Ameloblastoma
6	D	Cementoma

The most common odontogenic tumour is ameloblastoma, and this should be learnt comprehensively, as they crop up among the clinical cases.

4.22 Multiple Myeloma

1	D	60+ years
2	E	Male
3	H	African-Caribbean
4	M	Pepper pot skull
5	P	Plasma
6	Q	Bence Jones

Multiple myeloma is a fairly common cancer. It affects around 45 000 people in the USA at one time. There is increased prevalence in the African-Caribbean population. It accounts for around 1% of all cancers and 2% of all cancer deaths. It tends to occur more in men, especially if they have worked with petroleum. The classic findings are the pepper pot skull appearance in a skull X-ray and the presence of Bence Jones proteins in the urine. Patients tend to present with symptoms of hypercalcaemia. The treatment is usually pamidronate. Stem cell treatment is thought to benefit patients, however, it is not legal.

4.23 Syphilis

1 C *Treponema pallidum*

2 E Hutchinson

3 G Mulberry

4 J Snail track

5 L Gumma

6 M Aortic aneurysm

Treponema pallidum is the causative organism of syphilis, which is on the increase in the UK. It has an incubation period of between 9 and 90 days. In congenital syphilis, the malformations include frontal bossing, saddle nose, Hutchinson's incisors and Mulberry molars. Other problems include mental disability, deafness, sabre tibiae and Clutton's joints. In acquired syphilis the primary lesion is a chancre. This is a hard painless lesion that may ulcerate, and heals in 6–8 weeks. It is highly infectious. In secondary syphilis, snail track ulcers form. These are also highly infectious. In tertiary syphilis, a gumma forms in the midline of the palate or tongue. Gummas are not infectious and may be associated with aortic aneurysm or neurosyphilis.

4.24 Fibrous Dysplasia

1 C Equally prevalent in males and females

2 E 16–30 years

3 J Maxilla

4 L Ground glass

5 O Disfigurement and malocclusion

6 R No treatment, spontaneous arrest of progress with skeletal maturity

Fibrous dysplasia is seen in young adults and presents as a smooth and painless bony swelling of the maxilla. The swelling may disturb the occlusion. Radiographically it has a ground glass appearance. Typically there is spontaneous arrest of progress with skeletal maturity. Resection is only required when there is severe disfigurement or disturbed function.

4.25 Paget's Disease

1 C 50+ years

2 F 5%

3 J Pelvis

4 L Alkaline phosphatase

5 P Antibiotics

6 T 5 years

Paget's disease is radiographically detectable in 5% of the population; however, symptomatic disease is rarely found. The aetiology is unclear, but there is evidence of weak genetic and viral links. The condition is polyostotic and most frequently affects the pelvis, calvarium and limbs. The maxilla is occasionally affected, and the mandible is rarely affected. The initial lesions are predominantly osteolytic, but there is increasing sclerosis, often with generalised thickening of bone. Alkaline phosphatase levels are markedly raised. There is anarchic disorganisation of normal bone remodelling with characteristic alternating resorption and deposition. The osteoblastic action eventually prevails and produces thick bone that is susceptible to osteomyelitis. The disease is active for 3–5 years and then becomes static.

4.26 Kaposi's Sarcoma

1   A   Male

2   G   Human herpesvirus

3   D   HIV

4   K   Purple

5   M   Endothelial

6   R   2 years

Kaposi's sarcoma is caused by human herpesvirus 8. It is most commonly found in people with HIV infection. It is a purple plaque, and has three types: classic, endemic and epidemic. It is a tumour of the endothelial cells and is generally fatal within two years.

5
Oral Surgery

5.1 Theme: Facial Trauma Complications

5.2 Theme: Facial Trauma

5.3 Theme: Local Anaesthetics

5.4 Theme: Oro-Pharyngeal Anatomy

5.5 Theme: Complications of Extractions

5.6 Theme: Systemic Disease Affecting Exodontia

5.7 Theme: Neck Lumps

5.8 Theme: Sutures

5.9 Theme: Cranial Nerves

5.10 Theme: Nerve Injury

5.11 Theme: Parotid Diseases

5.12 Theme: Emergencies in the Dental Chair

5.13 Theme: Oral Lumps

5.14 Theme: Infection

5.15 Theme: Parotid Swelling

5.16 Theme: Extraction of Third Molars

5.17 Theme: Oral Cancer

5.18 Theme: Oro-Antral Fistula (1)

5.19 Theme: Oro-Antral Fistula (2)

5.20 Theme: Fractured Mandible - Epidemiology

5.21 Theme: Fractured Mandible

5.22 Theme: Fractured Orbital Floor

5.23 Theme: Non-Tumour Soft Tissue Lumps in the Mouth

5.24 Theme: Soft Tissue Lumps

5.25 Theme: Benign Tumours of the Mouth

5.26 Theme: Odontogenic Tumours

5.27 Theme: Anatomy (1)

5.28 Theme: Reconstruction using Free Flaps

5.29 Theme: Suture Materials

5.30 Theme: Post-operative Problems

5.31 Theme: Medication

5.32 Theme: Acute Trauma

5.33 Theme: Anatomy (2)

5.1 Theme: Facial Trauma Complications

A	Cavernous sinus thrombosis
B	Cerebral haemorrhage
C	Cerebrospinal fluid leakage
D	Base of skull fracture
E	Respiratory obstruction
F	Septal haematoma

For each of the following scenarios, choose the most likely complication from the list above. You may use each option once, more than once or not at all.

1. Clear watery nasal discharge.
2. Ophthalmoplegia may occur.
3. 'Panda eye' develops.
4. Retrograde infection of the facial veins.
5. Surgical airway may be lifesaving.

5.2 Theme: Facial Trauma

A	Malar/zygomatic arch fracture
B	Mandibular fracture
C	Maxillary fracture
D	Orbital blow-out fracture
E	Nasal fracture

For each of the following descriptions, choose the most appropriate option from the list above. You may use each option once, more than once or not at all.

1. Condylar neck is the weakest part.
2. Elevation is achieved by a temporal incision.
3. Extrusion of orbital contents into maxillary sinus may occur.
4. Le Fort described three different types.
5. Depressed cheek bone.
6. Step deformation of infraorbital ridge.

5.3 Theme: Local Anaesthetics

A   Articaine
B   Bupivacaine
C   Lignocaine
D   Mepivacaine
E   Prilocaine

For each of the following descriptions, choose the most appropriate option from the list above. You may use each option once, more than once or not at all.

1   0.5% concentration, 1:200,000 epinephrine, long duration of action.
2   4% concentration, 1:200,000 epinephrine, intermediate duration of action.
3   2% concentration, 1:80,000 epinephrine, intermediate duration of action.
4   3% concentration, felypressin, intermediate duration of action.
5   4% concentration, 1:100,000 epinephrine, intermediate duration of action.

5.4 Theme: Oro-Pharyngeal Anatomy

A   Epiglottic vallecula
B   Circumvallate papillae
C   Fovea palatini
D   Larynx
E   Nasopharynx
F   Oropharynx
G   Soft palate
H   Tonsil
I   Uvula
J   Vibrating line

For each of the following descriptions, choose the most appropriate anatomical feature from the list above. You may use each option once, more than once or not at all.

1   Lies between the tongue base and epiglottis and is common site for foreign body entrapment.
2   Conic projection from the posterior edge of the middle of the soft palate.
3   Dome-shaped structures on the human tongue that vary in number from eight to twelve.
4   Division between the movable and immovable tissues of the palate.
5   Eustachian tubes are located here.

5.5 Theme: Complications of Extractions

A	Buccal wall fracture
B	Damage to adjacent teeth
C	Mandibular fracture
D	Maxillary tuberosity fracture
E	Nerve damage
F	Oroantral communication
G	Oroantral fistula
H	Temporomandibular joint dislocation

For each of the following scenarios, select the most appropriate option from the list above. You may use each option once, more than once or not at all.

1. A patient returns after a difficult lower wisdom tooth extraction. He has a lateral open bite on the operative side and is dribbling. He complains of pain. On examination he is tender on the operative side, but there is no movement about the operative site.

2. A 28-year-old man is having his upper left third molar extracted. While elevating with a Cryer's, you see a tear in the palatal mucosa.

3. A 39-year-old woman complains of post-operative pain and 'whistling' 5 days after extraction of the upper left first molar by your principal. The socket is very large and full of debris.

5.6 Theme: Systemic Diseases Affecting Exodontia

A	Asthma	E	Lung cancer
B	Diabetes	F	Peripheral vascular disease
C	Epilepsy	G	Pituitary tumour
D	Human immunodeficiency virus (HIV) infection	H	Pregnancy

For each of the following scenarios, select the most appropriate option from the list above. You may use each option once, more than once or not at all.

1. A 65-year-old patient with this disease may well be on an anticoagulant, which will affect their management with regard to the timing of extraction with reference to INR.

2. In this group prilocaine (Citanest) with felypressin (Octapressin) should be avoided.

3. In this group, the patient should be well controlled before exodontia is attempted or referred to a specialist setting.

5.7 Theme: Neck Lumps

A   Brachial cyst
B   Cystic hygroma
C   Dermoid cyst
D   Graves' disease
E   Hashimoto's disease
F   Lymphoma
G   Ranula
H   Reactionary lymph node
I   Tuberculous lymph node
J   Thyroglossal cyst

For each of the following scenarios, select the most appropriate option from the list above. You may use each option once, more than once or not at all.

1. A 9-year-old child is brought to see you as the SHO in oral and maxillofacial surgery. He has a midline swelling, which moves on swallowing and protrusion of the tongue.

2. A 6-month-old child is referred to the department of oral and maxillofacial surgery. He has a solid, rubbery bilateral swelling, which has been present since birth. The lesion transilluminates brightly.

3. A 35-year-old man sees his GP as he is 'not feeling right'. He has been sweating at night, losing weight and has discomfort on drinking alcohol. On examination he has a large, rubbery lymph node on the right.

4. A woman presents with 'bulging' eyes, atrial fibrillation, weight loss and insomnia. On examination she has a tender enlarged midline swelling, which moves on swallowing.

5. A 21-year-old woman who has a recent history of acute pericoronitis is noted by her dentist to have a unilateral right submandibular region swelling.

5.8 Theme: Sutures

A 2/0 Black silk
B 8/0 nylon
C 3/0 Vicryl dyed
D 6/0 Prolene
E 3/0 nylon
F 3/0 Vicryl undyed
G 8/0 PDS
H 1/0 nylon

For each of the following scenarios, select the most appropriate option from the list above. You may use each option once, more than once or not at all.

1. The material of choice to close a mucoperiosteal envelope flap.
2. Your consultant asks you to close the thyroidectomy incision in layers with subcutaneous sutures to remove after 10 days.
3. The suture to hold a vacuum drain after submandibular gland excision.
4. A suture to close deep tissues on the face in the emergency department.
5. The suture used in microvascular anastomosis.

5.9 Theme: Cranial Nerves

A	I	H	VIII
B	II	I	IX
C	III	J	X
D	IV	K	XI
E	V	L	XII
F	VI	M	C2,C3
G	VII		

For each of the following questions, choose the most appropriate option from the list above. You may use each option once, more than once or not at all.

1. A patient presents with inability to smile and close their eye on the left side. Which nerve is responsible?
2. What other cranial nerve supply muscles of the facial region?
3. Which nerve is responsible for the movement of the intrinsic muscles of the tongue?
4. Which cranial nerve palsy is responsible for ptosis of the eyelid?
5. A patient complains of loss of sensation of the skin over the parotid region. Which nerve is responsible?

5.10 Theme: Nerve Injury

A   Facial nerve
B   Inferior alveolar nerve
C   Lingual nerve
D   5%
E   0.5%
F   2%
G   10%
H   Glossopharyngeal
I   Hypoglossal
J   1/200 000
K   0.05%
L   0.01%

For each of the following questions, choose the most appropriate option from the list above. You may use each option once, more than once or not at all.

1   What is the incidence of permanent lingual nerve injury subsequent to mandibular third molar surgery?

2   Which nerve neuropathy is most commonly idiopathic?

3   What is the incidence of temporary inferior alveolar nerve injury subsequent to mandibular third molar surgery?

4   A patient presents with deviation of the tongue on protrusion. Which nerve is responsible?

5   The patient presents with lack of sensation of their lower lip, gingivae and teeth on the right side. Which nerve is affected?

5.11 Theme: Parotid Diseases

A   Mumps
B   Measles virus
C   HIV virus
D   Coxsackie virus
E   Pleomorphic adenoma
F   Adenocarcinoma
G   Keratocyst
H   Adenoma
I   Salivary retention cyst
J   Salivary extravasation cyst
K   Salivary calculus
L   Gram-positive organisms
M   *Candida*

For each of the following questions, choose the most appropriate option from the list above. You may use each option once, more than once or not at all.

1. Which common childhood infection causes bilateral parotid enlargement?
2. Which salivary neoplasm is the most common in the parotid gland?
3. A patient presents with unilateral parotid swelling and facial palsy. What lesion would you suspect?
4. A patient presents with 'meal time syndrome'. What is your diagnosis?
5. A patient presents with pus exuding from Stensen's duct on the left side of their mouth. Which organism would you suspect?

ORAL SURGERY

5.12 Theme: Emergencies in the Dental Chair

A   Adrenaline 1:1000 (1 mg/ml)
B   Adrenaline 1:10 000 (1 mg/10 ml)
C   Aspirin oral
D   Chlorphenamine
E   Diazepam
F   Glucagon
G   Glucose
H   Glyceryl trinitrate spray
I   Hydrocortisone (IV)
J   Oxygen
K   Salbutamol

For each of the following scenarios, choose the most appropriate management option from the list above. You may use each option once, more than once or not at all.

1. Following oral administration of a 3 g sachet of amoxicillin, a 20-year-old woman reports shortness of breath and the development of a red rash over her body.

2. A 20-year-old man in your dental surgery waiting room is shaking involuntarily, frothing at the mouth and showing signs of incontinence.

3. A 57-year-old woman with type 1 diabetes collapses in the dental chair and a dipstick shows low blood glucose.

4. While being treated, a 60-year-old man complains of severe central crushing chest pain which radiates down the left arm and nausea. The pain does not respond to glyceryl trinitrate spray and oxygen.

5. A 30-year-old known asthmatic patient has just been told that she has to lose several of her teeth. She begins to wheeze and is short of breath.

5.13 Theme: Oral Lumps

A	Abscess	G	Kaposi's sarcoma
B	Adenoma	H	Metastatic lesion
C	Central giant cell granuloma	I	Mucocele
D	Fibroepithelial polyp	J	Peripheral giant cell granuloma
E	Gingival hyperplasia	K	Pyogenic granuloma
F	Haemangioma	L	Torus

For each of the following scenarios, choose the most appropriate diagnosis from the list above. You may use each option once, more than once or not at all.

1. Pregnant woman with a soft, red, fluctuant swelling on the gingiva.
2. Purple swelling of the hard palate that does not blanche on pressure in a young man.
3. A student with a pink swelling associated with multilocular radiolucency in the mandible.
4. Soft, well-circumscribed, pink swelling on the midline of the palate.
5. A sessile, fluctuant swelling on the lower lip, bluish in colour. There is history of trauma.

5.14 Theme: Infection

A	Candida albicans	F	Mycobacterium tuberculosis
B	Coxsackievirus	G	Staphylococcus aureus
C	Cytomegalovirus	H	Treponema pallidum
D	Epstein–Barr virus	I	Varicella zoster virus
E	Herpes simplex virus		

For each of the following soft tissue lesions, choose the most likely causative micro-organism from the list above. You may use each option once, more than once or not at all.

1. Multiple oral ulcers and fever in a child.
2. Multiple, unilateral ulcers in an elderly woman.
3. A single sinuous ulcer on the buccal mucosa of a 20-year-old.
4. White corrugated lesions found bilaterally on tongue in a young adult.
5. Multiple irregular ulcers on the soft tissue in an HIV-positive man.

5.15 Theme: Parotid Swelling

A	Acute parotitis
B	Adenocarcinoma
C	Bilateral salivary gland enlargement
D	Monomorphic adenoma
E	Mucoepidermoid carcinoma
F	Mumps
G	Pleomorphic adenoma
H	Polymorphous low-grade adenocarcinoma
I	Recurrent obstructive sialadenitis
J	Sarcoidosis
K	Tuberculosis
L	Wharton's tumour

For each of the following questions, choose the most appropriate option from the list above. You may use each option once, more than once or not at all.

1 Which of these pathologies is the most common benign tumour of the parotid gland?
2 What is a systemic cause of bilateral salivary gland enlargement?
3 Which condition is associated with Sjögren's disease?
4 Which condition is associated with Haerd Fort syndrome?
5 Which condition is associated with 'cold' abscesses?

ORAL SURGERY

5.16 Theme: Extraction of Third Molars

A   Impacted
B   Single episode of pericoronitis
C   Dentigerous cyst
D   Caries in distal adjacent second molar
E   Odontogenic keratocyst
F   Mandibular fracture
G   Radiotherapy
H   Pain
I   Periodontal disease of the second molar
J   Resorption of adjacent teeth
K   Inferior alveolar nerve neuropathy
L   Neoplasia
M   Acute infection (spreading)

For each of the following questions, choose the most appropriate option from the list above. You may use each option once, more than once or not at all.

1   Which recurrent multilocular lesion should be considered when assessing cysts associated with mandibular third molars?

2   What treatment is associated with osteoradionecrosis?

3   What lesions may be associated with resorption of adjacent second molar roots?

4   In what situation would you consider removal of a mandibular third molar after a single episode of pericoronitis?

5   If squamous cell carcinoma has developed in the lining of a dentigerous cyst associated with an impacted lower third molar, what symptom may the patient present with?

5.17 Theme: Oral Cancer

A Painful
B Painless
C Lymphadenopathy
D Mobile teeth
E Rolled borders
F Indurated
G Leukoplakia
H Neuropathy
I Trismus
J Alcohol
K Paan chewing
L Poor oral hygiene
M Smoking
N Age
O Trauma
P Tumour node metastasis (TNM)

For each of the following questions, choose the most appropriate option from the list above. You may use each option once, more than once or not at all.

1 What is the highest risk factor for oral cancer?
2 How do you classify the progression of a squamous cell carcinoma?
3 What symptom will imply involvement of masticatory muscles?
4 What symptom will imply involvement of nerves?
5 What is the second highest risk factor for oral cancer?

5.18 Theme: Oro-Antral Fistula (1)

A   Maxillary third permanent molar
B   Mandibular third permanent molar
C   Maxillary first permanent molar
D   Mandibular first permanent molar
E   Maxillary canine
F   Do not blow your nose
G   Rinse your mouth with warm salt mouthwashes four times a day
H   Use ice packs to reduce swelling of your face
I   Difficulty making dentures due to reduced sulcus depth
J   Paraesthesia/anaesthesia of the palate
K   Paraesthesia/anaesthesia of the upper lip
L   Paraesthesia of the posterior maxillary dentition
M   Unable to drink fluids without them bubbling through one's nose
N   Greater palatine nerve
O   Palatine artery
P   Palatal root of maxillary first permanent molar

For each of the following questions, choose the most appropriate option from the list above. You may use each option once, more than once or not at all.

1. Which tooth is most susceptible to oro-antral fistula?
2. What preventive advice should be given if you think a patient is at risk of an oro-antral fistula?
3. What is the most common complaint among patients who have an oro-antral fistula?
4. What is a common side-effect of a buccal advancement flap?
5. What anatomical structure should be avoided in a palatal rotation flap?

5.19 Theme: Oro-Antral Fistula (2)

A	An endothelium-lined connection between two endothelial surfaces
B	An epithelium-lined connection between two epithelial surfaces
C	Saline nasal spray
D	Ephedrine nasal spray
E	Atropine nasal spray
F	Dihydrocodeine tartrate
G	Aspirin
H	Ibuprofen
I	Cefuroxime
J	Amoxicillin
K	Metronidazole
L	Buccal pad of fat repair
M	Gillies lift
N	Sinus lift

For each of the following questions, choose the most appropriate option from the list above. You may use each option once, more than once or not at all.

1. What is the definition of a fistula?
2. Which nasal spray should be used in the pharmacological treatment of an oro-antral fistula?
3. Which analgesic should not be used in asthmatic people?
4. Which antibiotic is the drug of choice in treatment of an oro-antral fistula?
5. If initial treatment fails, which surgical procedure should be performed by an experienced clinician to attempt to close a persistent fistula?

5.20 Theme: Fractured Mandible – Epidemiology

A	Symphysis	G	Left
B	Parasymphysial	H	Right
C	Body	I	Interpersonal trauma
D	Angle	J	Pathological fracture
E	Condyle	K	Road traffic accident
F	Ramus	L	Sport-related injury

For each of the following questions, choose the most appropriate option from the list above. You may use each option once, more than once or not at all.

1. What is the most common site of a fracture in the mandible?
2. What is the second most common site of a fracture in the mandible?
3. Which side of the face do fractures occur most commonly?
4. What is the most common cause of a fractured mandible?
5. What was the most common cause of a fractured mandible 25 years ago?

5.21 Theme: Fractured Mandible

A	OCAR	I	Le Fort I
B	ORIF	J	Le Fort II
C	OTIM	K	Gunning
D	IMF	L	Markowitz
E	IPA	M	Patten
F	IRM	N	Inferior alveolar nerve
G	Bucket handle	O	Lingual nerve
H	Pan handle	P	Mylohyoid nerve

For each of the following questions, choose the most appropriate option from the list above. You may use each option once, more than once or not at all.

1. What is the acronym for the most common surgical treatment of a fractured mandible?
2. If a patient falls on their chin and sustains a bilateral parasymphysial fracture of the mandible, what is this called?
3. What is the name of the splint used to treat a fractured mandible in an edentulous patient?
4. What is the acronym used for the fixation of the mandible and maxilla together by wires?
5. Which nerve is most commonly injured when a patient sustains a fractured mandible?

5.22 Theme: Fractured Orbital Floor

- **A** Enophthalmos
- **B** Exophthalmos
- **C** Subconjunctival haemorrhage
- **D** Inferior rectus
- **E** Superior rectus
- **F** Lateral oblique
- **G** Inferior oblique
- **H** Diplopia
- **I** Retrobulbar haemorrhage
- **J** Step deformity
- **K** Detached retina
- **L** Hang drop sign
- **M** Swing shot sign

For each of the following questions, choose the most appropriate option from the list above. You may use each option once, more than once or not at all.

1. What is the most common symptom of a fractured orbital floor?
2. Which muscle is most commonly tethered in a fractured orbital floor?
3. What is the name for the sunken-in appearance of the eyeball?
4. What is the classic X-ray sign seen on an occipto-mental (OM) view in the case of an orbital floor fracture?
5. What medical emergency is associated with an orbital floor fracture?

5.23 Theme: Non-Tumour Soft Tissue Lumps in the Mouth

A	Basal cell carcinoma
B	Brown's tumour
C	Dermoid cyst
D	Epidermoid cyst
E	Fibroepithelial polyp
F	Mucocele
G	Mucoepidermoid cyst
H	Pyogenic granuloma
I	Ranula
J	Stafne's idiopathic bone cyst
K	Torus mandibularis
L	Torus palatinus

For each of the following descriptions, choose the most appropriate term from the list above. You may use each option once, more than once or not at all.

1. A giant cell lesion sometimes found in soft tissue but more commonly within bone. It occurs secondary to hyperparathyroidism, although the diagnosis is usually suggested after enucleation and histopathological examination which shows giant cells in a fibrous stroma.

2. A developmental cyst commonest at the lateral canthus of the eye, and next most often found in the midline of the neck above mylohyoid, where it causes elevation of the tongue.

3. A mucous extravasation cyst affecting the lower lip.

4. A cyst of the floor of the mouth arising from the sublingual gland. Tends to recur unless marsupialised. It can pass deep to mylohyoid and appears as a swelling in the neck and floor of mouth.

5. Bony lump found either in the centre of the palate.

5.24 Theme: Soft Tissue Lumps

A	Congenital epulis
B	Fibroepithelial polyp
C	Haemangioma
D	Lymphangioma
E	Peripheral giant cell granuloma
F	Pregnancy epulis
G	Pyogenic granuloma
H	Squamous cell carcinoma
I	Viral papillomata

For each of the following descriptions, choose the most appropriate term from the list above. You may use each option once, more than once or not at all.

1. By definition present at birth; usually presents as a pedunculated nodule. Histological examination reveals large granular cells.

2. A deep-red gingival swelling, probably caused by chronic irritation. Histological examination usually reveals a vascular lesion with multinucleated giant cells.

3. An increased inflammatory response to plaque during pregnancy causes a lesion indistinguishable from a pyogenic granuloma.

4. A red, fleshy swelling, often nodular, occurring as a response to recurrent trauma and non-specific infection. Histological examination shows proliferation of vascular connective tissue.

5. A lump that occurs as an over-vigorous response to recurrent trauma. It may be sessile or pedunculated, and presentation ranges from a small lump to lesions covering the entire palate.

5.25 Theme: Benign Tumours of the Mouth

A   Ameloblastoma
B   Fibroma
C   Granular cell myoblastoma
D   Lipoma
E   Neurofibroma
F   Neurolemmoma
G   Ossifying fibroma
H   Osteoma
I   Pindborg tumour
J   Squamous cell papilloma

For each of the following descriptions, choose the most appropriate term from the list above. You may use each option once, more than once or not at all.

1. Normally presents on the palate, is frequently cauliflower-shaped, and does not undergo malignant change.
2. A soft, smooth, slow growing, yellowish lump present in the cheek or neck.
3. A tumour comprised completely of Schwann cells.
4. A rare tumour of histiocytic origin which usually arises as a nodule on the tongue. Always excised with a margin.
5. May be a neoplasm or a developmental anomaly. It is a well-demarcated fibro-osseous lesion of the jaws. It presents as a painless, slow-growing swelling, expanding both buccal and lingual cortices. Similar histology to fibrous dysplasia.

5.26 Theme: Odontogenic Tumours

A Adenoameloblastoma
B Ameloblastic fibroma
C Ameloblastoma
D Calcifying epithelial odontogenic tumour
E Myxoma
F Odontome

For each of the following descriptions, choose the most appropriate term from the list above. You may use each option once, more than once or not at all.

1. Not a true neoplasm but a malformation of dental hard tissues. Classically, they are classified as compound, when they consist of multiple small 'teeth' in a fibrous sac, and complex, when they consist of a congealed, irregular mass of dental tissue.

2. Most common odontogenic tumour. Most common in men and Africans. Can be aggressive and invades surrounding tissue. Histologically there are two types seen: plexiform and follicular.

3. Characteristically seen as a radiolucency on X-ray with scattered radiopacities. Requires excision with a margin.

4. Can occur in both soft and hard tissues. Those arising in the jaws are tumours of the odontogenic mesenchyme. This tumour occurs in young men, arises within bone and has a soap bubble appearance on X-ray.

5. Rare tumour affecting young adults and appears as a unilocular radiolucency on X-ray causing painless expansion of the jaws. Enucleation is curative.

5.27 Theme: Anatomy (1)

A   Lateral pterygoid
B   Masseter
C   Medial pterygoid
D   Temporalis

For each of the following descriptions, choose the most appropriate muscle from the list above. You may use each option once, more than once or not at all.

1   Inserts on lateral surface of angle and lower ramus of mandible.
2   Inserts on the pterygoid fovea below condylar process of mandible and intra-articular cartilage of the temporomandibular joint.
3   Inserts on the medial and anterior aspect of coronoid process of mandible.
4   Action: elevates mandible and posterior fibres retract.
5   Action: elevates, protracts and laterally displaces mandible to opposite side for chewing.

5.28 Theme: Reconstruction using Free Flaps

A   Deep circumflex iliac flap
B   Deltopectoral flap
C   Fibula flap
D   Humerus flap
E   Latissimus dorsi flap
F   Masseter flap
G   Nasolabial flap
H   Pectoralis major flap
I   Radial forearm flap
J   Temporalis flap
K   Ulnar flap

For each of the following descriptions of flaps used for facial reconstruction in patients with oral cancer, choose the most appropriate name from the list above. You may use each option once, more than once or not at all.

1   Large bony flap, raised in close proximity to the common peroneal nerve.
2   Muscular flap of the face, raised and rotated into defects.
3   Fasciocutaneous flap. Raised from the forearm; blood supply from the ulnar artery must be checked otherwise problems with the hand may occur.
4   Very bulky flap based on thoracodorsal vessels. Needs to be tunnelled through axilla; can be raised as a free flap.
5   Can be used with or without bone. It is based on acromiothoracic vessels. Usually tunnelled after neck dissection.

5.29 Theme: Suture Materials

A	1/0 PDS
B	1/0 Prolene
C	1/0 Vicryl
D	3/0 Black silk
E	3/0 Prolene
F	3/0 Vicryl
G	5/0 Catgut
H	5/0 Prolene
I	5/0 Vicryl
J	9/0 Prolene
K	9/0 Stainless steel wire
L	9/0 Vicryl

For each of the following statements regarding suture materials, choose the most appropriate one from the list above. You may use each option once, more than once or not at all.

1. The correct material for arteriovenous anastomoses or vascular repair.
2. The traditional material of choice for suturing an apicoectomy incision.
3. The material of choice for suturing a skin biopsy in the infra-orbital region.
4. The material of choice for suturing deep (under the surface of the skin) in a skin wound.
5. Material that should not be used nowadays.

5.30 Theme: Post-operative Problems

A	Alveolar osteitis
B	Foreign body inhalation
D	Incorrect extraction
E	Infection
F	Ludwig's angina
G	Oral cancer
H	Osteomyelitis
I	Pneumonia
J	Retained root
K	Tuberculosis

For each of the following scenarios, choose the most appropriate diagnosis from the list above. You may use each option once, more than once or not at all.

1 A patient presents at your surgery 2 days after a very routine extraction, complaining of pain in the same site where the tooth was extracted. The patient complains that the pain is much worse than the original toothache. On examination the patient is apyrexic and there is food debris in the socket.

2 A patient presents a month after a routine extraction complaining of a bad taste in their mouth coming from the extraction site, but no pain. On examination the socket has not healed entirely, and there is mild swelling in the region.

3 A patient presents to your surgery a week after extraction of four wisdom teeth, looking very unwell and pyrexic. The patient has difficulty talking, trismus and bilateral drooling. On examination, the tongue is raised towards the roof of the mouth.

4 An elderly patient has had open reduction and internal fixation of the mandible following a fall. One week later she has shortness of breath and associated pyrexia. She is confused.

5 A 65-year-old patient presents 2 months after extraction of two mobile teeth. He complains of non-healing sockets which breakdown and bleed. On examination, the patient has bilateral lymphadenopathy. The X-ray shows no retained roots, but an unusual appearance of the bone.

ORAL SURGERY

5.31 Theme: Medication

A	3 g amoxicillin PO 1 hour pre-op	I	500 mg
B	2 g amoxicillin PO 1 hour pre-op	J	400 mg
C	1.5 g amoxicillin PO 1 hour pre-op	K	250 mg
D	900 mg clindamycin PO 1 hour pre-op	L	Four times daily
E	600 mg clindamycin PO 1 hour pre-op	M	Three times daily
F	300 mg clindamycin PO 1 hour pre-op	N	Twice daily
G	Erythromycin		
H	Metronidazole		

For each of the following statements, choose the most appropriate option from the list above. You may use each option once, more than once or not at all.

1 A 10-year-old with no allergies requiring antibiotic cover.
2 A 40-year-old man requires antibiotic cover. He has been treated with penicillin 2 weeks ago.
3 The drug of choice for a dental abscess.
4 The dose of choice of ibuprofen.
5 The frequency of dose of ibuprofen per day.

5.32 Theme: Acute Trauma

A Airway
B Breathing
C Circulation
D Disability
E Exposure
F Radiographic review

For each of the following stages of the primary survey, choose the most appropriate name from the list above. You may use each option once, more than once or not at all.

1 First
2 Second
3 Third
4 Fourth
5 Fifth

5.33 Theme: Anatomy (2)

A Articular eminence
B Condylar head
C Glenoid fossa
D Lateral ligament
E Meniscus
F Sphenomandibular ligament
G Stylomandibular ligament

For each of the blanks in the following statements, choose the most appropriate option from the list above. You may use each option once, more than once or not at all.

1 The ………. passes from the sphenoid bone to the lingula next to the inferior dental canal.

2 The ………. arises from the styloid process and is attached to the angle of the mandible.

3 The temporomandibular joint has a fibrous capsule which is attached to the articular margins. The lateral part of the capsule is thickened to form the …………

4 The joint cavity is divided into two by a disc of dense fibrous connective tissue. It is called the ………… .

5 The upper cavity of the joint is long and includes both a concave surface of the temporal bone and a convex bulge on the underside of the zygomatic arch. The latter bulge is called the ………… .

5.1 Facial Trauma Complications

1	C	Cerebrospinal fluid leakage
2	A	Cavernous sinus thrombosis
3	D	Base of skull fracture
4	A	Cavernous sinus thrombosis
5	E	Respiratory obstruction

Clear watery nasal discharge is sign of cerebrospinal fluid leakage or rhinorrhea after facial trauma, as perforation into the anterior cranial fossa can cause a communication and hence leakage.

Ophthalmoplegia is a paralysis or weakness of one or more of the muscles that control eye movement. A tumour, aneurysm or thrombosis in the cavernous sinus, located behind the eyes, can cause painful ophthalmoplegia as well as thyroid disease, diabetes mellitus, brainstem tumours, migraine, basilar artery stroke, pituitary stroke, myasthenia gravis, muscular dystrophy, and the Fisher variant of Guillain–Barré syndrome.

Panda eyes or raccoon eyes (USA), periorbital ecchymosis, is a sign of a base of skull fracture or subgaleal haematoma, a craniotomy that ruptured the meninges, or (rarely) certain cancers. This sign is late following trauma.

The danger triangle of the face consists of the area from the corners of the mouth to the bridge of the nose, including the nose and maxilla. Due to the special nature of the blood supply to the human nose and surrounding area, it is possible for retrograde infections from the nasal area to spread to the brain causing cavernous sinus thrombosis, meningitis or brain abscess.

Respiratory obstruction if not dislodging after the Heimlich manoeuvre may require an emergency surgical airway, i.e. cricothyroidotomy then converted to a tracheostomy.

5.2 Facial Trauma

1 B Mandibular fracture

2 A Malar/zygomatic arch fracture

3 D Orbital blow-out

4 C Maxillary fracture

5 A Malar fracture

6 A Malar fracture

Condylar neck is the weakest part of the mandible and can fracture easily with trauma. The zygoma or malar is elevated by a temporal incision. Step deformities on the infra-orbital ridge, depression of the cheek and a step over the fronto-zygomatico suture can indicate a zygomatic fracture. The fat in the floor of the orbit can herniate into the fracture site and cause restriction of the inferior rectus muscle.

The Le Fort classification comprises the following types.

Le Fort type 1

- Horizontal maxillary fracture, separating the teeth from the upper face
- Fracture line passes through the alveolar ridge, lateral nose and inferior wall of maxillary sinus

Le Fort type 2

- Pyramidal fracture, with the teeth at the pyramid base, and nasofrontal suture at its apex
- Fracture arch passes through posterior alveolar ridge, lateral walls of maxillary sinuses, inferior orbital rim and nasal bones

Le Fort type 3

- Craniofacial disjunction
- Fracture line passes through naso-frontal suture, maxillo-frontal suture, orbital wall and zygomatic arch

5.3 Local Anaesthetics

1 B Bupivacaine

2 A Articaine

3 C Lignocaine

4 E Prilocaine

5 A Articaine

Levobupivacaine is also available at 0.5% concentration with 1:200,000 epinephrine; it is long acting with reported lower toxicity compared to bupivacaine.

5.4 Oro-Pharyngeal Anatomy

1. A Epiglottic vallecula

2. I Uvula

3. B Circumvallate papillae

4. J Vibrating line

5. E Nasopharynx

The epiglottic vallecula is a depression ('vallecula') just behind the root of the tongue between the folds in the throat. These depressions serve as 'spit traps'; saliva is temporarily held in the vallecula to prevent initiation of the swallowing reflex.

Circumvallate papillae are situated on the surface of the tongue immediately in front of the foramen cecum and sulcus terminalis, forming a row on either side; the two rows run backward and medially, and meet in the midline.

The fovea palatini consists of two small depressions in the posterior aspect of the palate, one on each side of the midline, at or near the attachment of the soft palate to the hard palate.

The larynx, commonly called the voice box, produces pitch and volume. The larynx houses the vocal folds (vocal cords), which are essential for phonation. The vocal folds are situated just below where the tract of the pharynx splits into the trachea and the oesophagus.

The upper portion of the pharynx, the nasopharynx, extends from the base of the skull to the upper surface of the soft palate.

The oropharynx lies behind the oral cavity, extending from the uvula to the level of the hyoid bone.

The tonsils are collections of lymphoid tissue facing into the aerodigestive tract. The palatine tonsils and the nasopharyngeal tonsils are located near the oropharynx and nasopharynx (parts of the throat).

ORAL SURGERY

5.5 Complications of Extractions

1 H Temporomandibular joint dislocation

There is no movement about the extraction site, so it is not a fracture, but poor technique in supporting the mandible during extractions can lead to dislocations.

2 D Maxillary tuberosity fracture

The palatal split occurs as you have fractured the maxillary tuberosity and is a good sign for you to stop and rethink. If you have your hands properly in place to support this region, you will feel the bone giving and hopefully stop elevating before you fracture the bone.

3 F Oroantral communication

This woman has an oroantral communication and not an oroantral fistula, as there has not been long enough for the communication to epithelialise, which takes 10–14 days.

5.6 Systemic Diseases Affecting Exodontia

1 F Peripheral vascular disease

Peripheral vascular disease patients are often on warfarin, although the therapeutic range is lower.

2 H Pregnancy

Pregnancy in the third trimester is a contraindication to this anaesthetic agent, as felypressin may lead to labour.

3 C Epilepsy

Patients with poorly controlled epilepsy should not have exodontia under local anaesthesia, as they are prone to fits. The extraction should be delayed until they are stable or they can be referred for extraction under sedation.

5.7 Neck Lumps

1 J Thyroglossal cyst

2 B Cystic hygroma

3 F Lymphoma

4 D Graves' disease

5 H Reactionary lymph node

Thyroglossal duct cysts present as a midline neck lump that is usually painless, smooth and cystic; if infected, pain can occur. There may be difficulty breathing, difficulty swallowing, and discomfort in the upper abdomen, especially if the lump becomes large. Cystic hygroma is a congenital multiloculated lymphatic lesion that can arise anywhere, but is classically found in the neck. This is the most common form of lymphangioma. It consists of large, cyst-like cavities containing watery fluid. Lymphoma frequently presents with night sweats and lymphadenopathy.

5.8 Sutures

1 C 3/0 Vicryl dyed

2 E 3/0 nylon

3 A 2/0 Black silk

4 F 3/0 Vicryl undyed

5 B 8/0 nylon

The ideal suture has the following characteristics:

- It is sterile.
- It is all-purpose (composed of material that can be used in any surgical procedure).
- It causes minimal tissue injury or tissue reaction (ie, non-electrolytic, non-capillary, non-allergenic, non-carcinogenic).
- It is easy to handle.
- It holds securely when knotted (ie, no fraying or cutting).
- It has high tensile strength.
- It has a favourable absorption profile.
- It is resistant to infection.

5.9 Cranial Nerves

1 G VII

2 E V

3 L XII

4 C III

5 M C2,C3

If a student is unable to correlate cranial nerves with a clinical scenario, it does not create a good impression, as this should have been learnt in the preclinical years.

5.10 Nerve Injury

1 E 0.5%

2 A Facial nerve

3 F 2%

4 I Hypoglossal

5 B Inferior alveolar nerve

Nerve injury is a common and serious side-effect of wisdom tooth extraction. The correct statistics should be quoted to a patient when taking consent, to make sure that the consenting procedure is valid.

5.11 Parotid Diseases

1 A Mumps

2 E Pleomorphic adenoma

3 F Adenocarcinoma

4 K Salivary calculus

5 L Gram-positive organisms

Students should be able to differentiate between symptoms which are serious and symptoms which are less serious.

5.12 Emergencies in the Dental Chair

1 A Adrenaline 1:1000 (1 mg/ml)

2 E Diazepam

3 F Glucagon

4 C Aspirin oral

5 K Salbutamol

Treatment of medical emergencies is a pass/fail topic and should be known inside out.

5.13 Oral Lumps

1 K Pyogenic granuloma

2 G Kaposi's sarcoma

3 J Peripheral giant cell granuloma

4 L Torus

5 I Mucocele

Mucoceles are generally excised; however, if the cause is not removed (parafunction such as lip biting or poor restoration), this may recur.

Tori rarely need removal, unless they prevent seating of a denture. Kaposi's sarcoma is associated with human herpesvirus and HIV.

5.14 Infection

1 E Herpes simplex virus

2 I Varicella zoster virus

3 H *Treponema pallidum*

4 D Epstein-Barr virus

5 C Cytomegalovirus

The above lesions are common presentations of bacterial and viral infections. Primary herpetic gingivostomatitis in children is often mistaken for teething. The treatment is analgesia and fluid support. The presence of unilateral lesions on the face is the classic presentation of herpes zoster.

5.15 Parotid Swelling

1	G	Pleomorphic adenoma
2	F	Mumps
3	I	Recurrent obstructive sialadenitis
4	J	Sarcoidosis
5	K	Tuberculosis

Mumps causes the classic bilateral parotitis, but it can present as a unilateral enlargement in rare cases. Haerd Fort syndrome includes sarcoidosis. Tuberculosis historically was associated with 'cold abscesses'. It is caused by *Mycobacterium tuberculosis*, an acid-fast bacterium that does not stain with Gram stain. It requires Ziehl–Nielsen staining.

5.16 Extraction of Third Molars

1	E	Odontogenic keratocyst
2	G	Radiotherapy
3	J	Resorption of adjacent teeth
4	M	Acute infection (spreading)
5	K	Inferior alveolar nerve neuropathy

An odontogenic keratocyst is usually multilocular. Wisdom teeth should only be extracted if there have been two episodes of pericoronitis or one severe episode with spreading infection.

5.17 Oral Cancer

1 K Paan chewing

2 P TNM

3 I Trismus

4 H Neuropathy

5 M Smoking

Knowing the epidemiology of oral cancer is important. When you assess a patient, it is not just the lesion but also the risk factors present which give you the diagnosis. It is important to ask if the patient smokes and also if the patient ever smoked, for how long and how many cigarettes per day?

5.18 Oro-Antral Fistula (1)

1 C Maxillary first permanent molar

2 F Do not blow your nose

3 M Unable to drink fluids without them bubbling through one's nose

4 I Difficulty making dentures due to reduced sulcus depth

5 O Palatine artery

The teeth which are at greatest risk of an oro-antral fistula are the maxillary first permanent molars, as they are in close proximity to the antrum. It is important to tell patients not to blow their nose as the pressure can damage the initial healing that occurs in up to 95% of oro-antral fistulas. As dentists we only see oro-antral fistulas either when they are enormous initially (and will not close without the intervention of a second procedure, often done best immediately) or when a patient presents with secondary symptoms. The only downside to a buccal advancement flap is that it reduces sulcus depth. However, it is a simple procedure that most dentists should be able to perform, and it is very successful.

ORAL SURGERY

5.19 Oro-Antral Fistula (2)

1	B	An epithelium-lined connection between two epithelial surfaces
2	D	Ephedrine nasal spray
3	H	Ibuprofen
4	I	Cefuroxime
5	L	Buccal pad of fat repair

Ibuprofen is contraindicated in asthmatic people. Cefuroxime is the most efficacious drug in this scenario, as it has the broadest antimicrobial coverage. The buccal pad of fat repair is an operation with a very good success rate, but should only be performed by experienced clinicians.

5.20 Fractured Mandible – Epidemiology

1	D	Angle
2	E	Condyle
3	G	Left
4	I	Interpersonal trauma
5	K	Road traffic accident

Fractured mandibles occur mainly among 16–25-year-old males. Most people are right handed and therefore when trying to hit someone else, they make contact with the left side of the face. The most common cause in England is interpersonal trauma. The Seatbelt Act 1983 brought about a massive reduction in the number of mandibles fractured in road traffic accidents. In Asia and Africa it is still the number one cause of a fractured mandible.

5.21 Fractured Mandible

1 B ORIF

2 G Bucket handle

3 K Gunning

4 D IMF

5 N Inferior alveolar nerve

The most common way of surgically treating a fractured mandible is by open reduction internal fixation (ORIF). Fixing the mandible and maxilla together is done by inter-maxillary fixation (IMF). A bucket-handle fracture is a bilateral parasymphysial fracture. A Gunning splint is either a custom-made device or the patient's own dentures are customised by removing all the canines and incisors. The dentures are wired into the maxilla and mandible and then wired together. The most common nerve to be injured is the inferior alveolar nerve.

5.22 Fractured Orbital Floor

1 H Diplopia

2 D Inferior rectus

3 A Enophthalmos

4 L Hang drop sign

5 I Retrobulbar haemorrhage

Enophthalmos and subconjunctival haemorrhage are the most common signs of a fractured orbital floor; however, the most common symptom is diplopia. There are three main causes of diplopia in a fractured orbital floor:

- The eyeball is sunken in places so it is out of synchrony with the other eyeball.
- An intrinsic muscle of the eyeball (most commonly the lateral rectus) is tethered on a fracture fragment, preventing movement of the eyeball.

ORAL SURGERY

- Rarely there is neuronal damage to one of the intrinsic muscles of the eyeball.

The classic sign on an OM radiograph is the hang drop sign, illustrating the herniation of the orbital fat pad through the fracture. The medical emergency here is a retrobulbar haemorrhage (bleeding behind the globe of the eye). The patient presents with a painful proptosed eye and needs emergency surgical drainage and arrest of the bleed, otherwise blindness results.

5.23 Non-Tumour Soft Tissue Lumps in the Mouth

1 B Brown's tumour

2 C Dermoid cyst

3 F Mucocele

4 I Ranula

5 L Torus palatinus

Ranula is Greek for frog. A ranula gives the appearance of a frog's neck. It can pass through mylohyoid and transilluminates. It tends to appear in children.

5.24 Soft Tissue Lumps

1 A Congenital epulis

2 E Peripheral giant cell granuloma

3 F Pregnancy epulis

4 G Pyogenic granuloma

5 B Fibroepithelial polyp

Soft tissue lumps need to be differentiated into what is suspicious and what is not. However, if unsure of the diagnosis, it is always best to refer for clarification.

5.25 Benign Tumours of the Mouth

1 J Squamous cell papilloma

2 D Lipoma

3 F Neurolemmoma

4 C Granular cell myoblastoma

5 G Ossifying fibroma

These are generally unusual conditions, but some of the 'classic' descriptions can be used to identify these lesions.

5.26 Odontogenic Tumours

1 F Odontome

2 C Ameloblastoma

3 D Calcifying epithelial odontogenic tumour

4 E Myxoma

5 B Ameloblastic fibroma

Ameloblastoma is the most common odontogenic malignancy found in the mouth. It is important to diagnose it early otherwise it can lead to considerable destruction of the mandible.

ORAL SURGERY

5.27 Anatomy (1)

1 B Masseter

2 A Lateral pterygoid

3 D Temporalis

4 D Temporalis

5 C Medial pterygoid

It is important to know your anatomy, especially the simplest things such as the muscles of mastication.

5.28 Reconstruction using Free Flaps

1 C Fibula flap

2 J Temporalis flap

3 I Radial forearm flap

4 E Latissimus dorsi flap

5 E Latissimus dorsi flap

When describing oral cancer it is useful to be able to talk about some of the reconstructive methods to impress examiners!

5.29 Suture Materials

1 J 9/0 Prolene

2 D 3/0 Black silk

3 H 5/0 Prolene

4 F 3/0 Vicryl

5 G 5/0 Catgut

Suture materials are either resorbable or non-resorbable. The main resorbable materials are Vicryl and Ethilon. The non-resorbable materials are Prolene, PDS and black silk. Stainless steel is used in thoracic surgery and not really in maxillofacial surgery. Catgut sutures are no longer in production in the UK, as there is a risk of bovine spongiform encephalopathy. The smaller the number next to the suture (e.g. 1/0), the thicker the material. 9/0 is extremely fine and a magnifying microscope is needed when using it.

5.30 Post-operative Problems

1 A Alveolar osteitis

2 J Retained root

3 F Ludwig's angina

4 I Pneumonia

5 G Oral cancer

Infection usually takes a few days to occur, so if the patient re-presents in the first couple of days, an infection is likely. The most common complication of extraction is alveolar osteitis. The elderly inpatient in Q 4 illustrates the fact that not all problems are of dental origin. A bed-bound patient who is pyrexic and confused may well have pneumonia, especially of they are short of breath and pyrexic as well. Ludwig's angina is a medical emergency, associated with significant mortality. These patients need to be treated in hospital as an acute emergency. A patient with a non-healing socket should be treated with suspicion. The three main diagnoses are retained root, osteomyelitis and oral cancer.

ORAL SURGERY

5.31 Medication

1	C	1.5 g amoxicillin PO 1 hour pre-op
2	E	600 mg clindamycin PO 1 hour pre-op
3	H	Metronidazole
4	J	400 mg
5	M	Three times daily

The 10-year-old should have half the dose of an adult. Metronidazole is the drug of choice for dental infections. Ibuprofen should be given 400 mg three times daily for five days.

5.32 Acute Trauma

1	A	Airway
2	B	Breathing
3	C	Circulation
4	D	Disability
5	E	Exposure

The first stage of the primary survey in acute trauma is to establish a patent airway and protect the cervical spine from any further injury. Then assess the breathing and circulation. Count the respiratory rate. Give 100% oxygen.

- Circulation with haemorrhage control – assess the level of consciousness, skin colour, pulse and blood pressure, manual pressure control of major haemorrhage. Establish two large venous lines, cannulae, take blood for cross-match and baseline studies.
- Disability – use AVPU: is the patient *a*lert, responding to *v*ocal stimuli, responding to *p*ainful stimuli or *u*nresponsive.
- Exposure – remove all clothing to establish the extent of all injuries.

ANSWERS

5.33 Anatomy (2)

1 F Sphenomandibular ligament

2 G Stylomandibular ligament

3 D Lateral ligament

4 E Meniscus

5 A Articular eminence

6 Periodontics

6.1 Theme: Syndromes associated with Gingival Overgrowth

6.2 Theme: Gracey Curettes

6.3 Theme: Local Drug Delivery in the Management of Periodontal Diseases

6.4 Theme: Periodontitis as a Manifestation of Systemic Disease

6.5 Theme: Systemic Diseases associated with Periodontal Disease

6.6 Theme: Micro-organisms

6.7 Theme: Plaque, Pellicle, Gingivitis and Calculus

6.8 Theme: Risk Factors

6.9 Theme: Basic Periodontal Examination (BPE)

6.10 Theme: Acute Necrotising Ulcerative Gingivitis (ANUG)

6.11 Theme: Juvenile Periodontitis – Epidemiology

6.12 Theme: Juvenile Periodontitis

6.13 Theme: Lateral Periodontal Abscess

6.14 Theme: Drugs and Periodontal Disease

6.15 Theme: Treatment Options and the BPE

6.16 Theme: Curettage

6.17 Theme: Periodontal Probes

6.18 Theme: Down Syndrome

6.19 Theme: Gingivostomatitis

6.20 Theme: Gram Staining

6.21 Theme: Papillon-Lefèvre Disease

6.22 Theme: Immunoglobulins

6.23 Theme: Diabetes

6.24 Theme: Topical Antimicrobials

6.25 Theme: Indices

6.26 Theme: Periodontal Instruments

PERIODONTICS

6.1 Theme: Syndromes associated with Gingival Overgrowth

A	Apert
B	Chediak–Higashi
C	Cross
D	Laband
E	Ramon
F	Rutherfurd
G	Turner

For each of the descriptions below, choose the most likely syndrome associated with gingival fibromatosis from the list of options above. Each option may be used once, more than once or not at all.

1. Abnormal nasal morphology, macrotia, delayed tooth eruption and gingival fibromatosis.
2. Anonychia, hypertrichosis, delayed tooth eruption and gingival fibromatosis.
3. Athetosis, learning disability, hypopigmentation and gingival fibromatosis.
4. Cherubism, hypertrichosis, epilepsy and gingival fibromatosis.
5. Corneal dystrophy, hearing loss, delayed tooth eruption and gingival fibromatosis.

6.2 Theme: Gracey Curettes

A	1/2	F	11/12
B	3/4	G	13/14
C	5/6	H	15/16
D	7/8	I	17/18
E	9/10		

From the Gracey curette instrument numbers listed above, choose the one which would be best indicated for root surface debridement of the teeth surfaces listed below. You may use each option once, more than once or not at all.

1. Buccal surface of the maxillary second premolar
2. Distal surface of the mandibular first premolar
3. Distal surface of the maxillary third molar
4. Lingual surface of maxillary first premolar
5. Mesial surface of the mandibular second molar

PERIODONTICS

6.3 Theme: Local Drug Delivery in the Management of Periodontal Diseases

A	Azithromycin
B	Chlorhexidine
C	Doxycycline
D	Metronidazole
E	Minocycline
F	Tetracycline

From the option list above of active ingredients, match with the correct proprietary brand below. You may use each option once, more than once or not at all.

1. Arestin
2. Atridox
3. Elyzol
4. PerioChip
5. Periocline

6.4 Theme: Periodontitis as a Manifestation of Systemic Disease

A	Asperger syndrome
B	Chediak–Higashi syndrome
C	Cohen syndrome
D	Down syndrome
E	Ehlers–Danlos syndrome
F	Familial neutropenia
G	Histiocytosis syndrome
H	Hypophosphatasia
I	Papillon–Lefèvre syndrome

For the following clinical scenarios, choose the most appropriate diagnosis from the list above. You may use each option once, more than once or not at all.

1. Caused by trisomy of chromosome 21.
2. Hyperkeratosis of the feet and hands.
3. Abnormal increase in histiocytes.
4. Defective bone and tooth mineralisation.
5. Double-jointedness, easily bruised with vision problems.

6.5 Theme: Systemic Diseases associated with Periodontal Disease

A	Chediak-Higashi syndrome
B	Cohen syndrome
C	Down syndrome
D	Ehlers-Danlos syndrome (types IV and VIII)
E	Familial and cyclic neutropenia
F	Glycogen storage disease
G	Histiocytosis syndrome
H	Hypophosphatasia
I	Leukocyte adhesion deficiency syndromes
J	Papillon-Lefèvre syndrome

For each of the following scenarios, choose the best option from the list above. You may use each option once, more than once or not at all.

1 A syndrome that is due to an autosomal recessive disorder, arising from a mutation in the lysosomal trafficking regulator gene LYST. It particularly affects the immune system with persistent infections.

2 A syndrome associated with the presence of all or part of an extra chromosome 21. It is estimated to occur in 1 per 800–1000 births. It is associated with microgenia, macroglossia and increased risk of periodontal disease.

3 A syndrome typically thought of as a cancer-like condition. It is thought to affect roughly 1 in 200,000 people each year. It may also be referred to as pulmonary Langerhans cell granulomatosis.

4 A syndrome that is an autosomal recessive genetic disorder caused by a deficiency in cathepsin C. It is characterised by periodontitis and palmoplantar keratoderma.

6.6 Theme: Micro-organisms

A   *Actinobacillus actinomycetemcomitans*
B   *Actinomyces israelii*
C   *Borrelia vincentii*
D   *Candida albicans*
E   *Lactobacillus*
F   *Porphyromonas gingivalis*
G   *Treponema pallidum*
H   *Streptococcus milleri*
I   *Streptococcus mutans*
J   *Streptococcus salivarius*
K   *Streptococcus sanguis*

For each of the following statements, choose the most appropriate option from the list above. You may use each option once, more than once or not at all.

1   Aerobic; synthesises dextran. Colony density rises to > 50% in presence of high dietary sucrose. Able to produce acid from most sugars. The most important bacterium in the aetiology of dental caries.

2   Accounts for half the streptococci in plaque and is strongly implicated in half the cases of subacute bacterial endocarditis.

3   Secondary coloniser in caries (mainly dentine).

4   Obligate anaerobe. A member of the 'black pigmented' *Bacteroides* group, which is associated with rapidly progressive periodontitis.

5   A spirochaete which causes syphilis.

6   Yeast-like fungus, famous as an opportunistic oral pathogen, probably carried as a commensal by most people.

7   Filamentous organism, implicated in root caries. Can cause a rare persistent infection of the jaws, mouth and female reproductive system.

8   Microaerophilic Gram-negative rod. Found particularly in juvenile periodontitis and rapidly progressive periodontitis.

9   Commonly isolated from dental abscesses, also implicated in abscess formation at other sites in the body.

10 The largest oral spirochaete.

6.7 Theme: Plaque, Pellicle, Gingivitis and Calculus

A 20%
B 40%
C 60%
D 80%
E Spirochaetes
F Streptococci
G *Actinomyces*
H Obligate anaerobes
I Gram-positive bacteria
J Gram-negative bacteria

For each of the following questions, choose the most appropriate option from the list above. You may use each option once, more than once or not at all.

1 Which bacteria first colonise plaque after 3-4 hours?
2 After 10-12 days which bacteria predominate in gingivitis?
3 Which group of bacteria predominate in subgingival plaque?
4 Which group of bacteria predominate in supragingival plaque?
5 What percentage of calculus is made up of inorganic salts?

6.8 Theme: Risk Factors

A Acute bleeding
B Acute necrotising ulcerative gingivitis (ANUG)
C Epulis
D Hyperplasia
E Periodontal disease of the deciduous dentition

For each of the following conditions and risk factors, choose the most appropriate periodontal condition from the list above. You may use each option once, more than once or not at all.

1 Pregnancy
2 Smoking
3 Acute leukaemia
4 Renal transplant
5 Chediak–Higashi disease

6.9 Theme: Basic Periodontal Examination (BPE)

A 0
B 1
C 2
D 3
E 4
F 5
G 6

For each of the following scenarios, choose the most appropriate BPE score from the list above. You may use each option once, more than once or not at all.

1. The black band of the World Health Organization (WHO) probe is not visible.
2. There is a plaque-retentive factor but no pocket.
3. Some but not all of the black band of the WHO probe is visible.
4. The whole of the black band of the WHO probe is visible but there is a pocket present.
5. There is gingival bleeding but no pocketing.

6.10 Theme: Acute Necrotising Ulcerative Gingivitis (ANUG)

A	Europe	Q	Target lesion
B	Asia	R	Circumvallate
C	South America	S	Punched out
D	Africa	T	Antibiotics only
E	Streptococci	U	Antibiotics and mouthwash
F	Spirochaetes	V	Debridement, antibiotics and mouthwash
G	*Actinobacillus actinomycetemcomitans*	W	Metronidazole
H	Staphylococci	X	Amoxicillin
I	Oral cancer	Y	Erythromycin
J	Cancrum oris	Z	Under 25 years
K	Actinomycosis	AA	25–40 years
L	AIDS	BB	40+ years
M	Chediak–Higashi disease	CC	Chlorhexidine
N	Leukaemia	DD	Sodium perborate
O	Male	EE	Peroxyl
P	Female		

For each of the following questions, choose the most appropriate option from the list above. You may use each option once, more than once or not at all.

1. Which area of the world does ANUG occur in?
2. What disease can it lead to, if left unchecked?
3. Which bacteria mainly cause it?
4. Which age group does it mainly affect?
5. Which sex does it affect predominantly?
6. What is the characteristic description of the ulceration on the gingivae?
7. What is the treatment of choice?
8. Which mouthwash should be prescribed?
9. Which antibiotic should be prescribed?
10. If the patient has lymphadenopathy, which systemic disorder should be considered?

6.11 Theme: Juvenile Periodontitis – Epidemiology

A 0.01%
B 0.05%
C 0.1%
D 0.5%
E 1%
F 5%
G American
H Asian
I Black
J Scandinavian
K Male
L Female
M Average
N Good
O Poor

For each of the following questions, choose the most appropriate option from the list above. You may use each option once, more than once or not at all.

1. Localised juvenile periodontitis affects what proportion of the population?
2. Generalised juvenile periodontitis affects what proportion of the population?
3. Which ethnic group does it most commonly occur in?
4. Which sex does it occur in more frequently?
5. What is the oral hygiene like in these patients?

6.12 Theme: Juvenile Periodontitis

A	Canines	I	Complement function
B	Molars	J	Lymphocyte function
C	Incisors	K	Neutrophil chemotaxis
D	Premolars	L	Erythromycin
E	*Actinomyces actinomycetemcomitans*	M	Penicillin
F	Leptospira	N	Tetracycline
G	Spirochaetes		
H	Streptococci		

For each of the following questions, choose the most appropriate option from the list above. You may use each option once, more than once or not at all.

1 Which teeth does it affect first?
2 Which teeth does it affect next?
3 Which bacterium causes it?
4 What defect may be present in the patient's immune system?
5 Which antibiotic is the drug of choice for this condition?

6.13 Theme: Lateral Periodontal Abscess

A	No pain	I	Non-vital
B	Pain	J	Vital
C	Sensitive to apical percussion	K	Widened periodontal ligament
D	Not sensitive to percussion	L	Vertical bone loss
E	Sensitive to lateral percussion	M	Horizontal bone loss
F	No pocketing		
G	Sometimes pocketing		
H	Always pocketing		

For each of the following areas, choose the most appropriate finding from the list above for a patient who has a lateral periodontal abscess. You may use each option once, more than once or not at all.

1 History
2 Percussion
3 Probing
4 Vitality
5 X-ray

PERIODONTICS

6.14 Theme: Drugs and Periodontal Disease

A Anti-inflammatory
B Antibiotic
C Chemotherapeutic drug
D Epilepsy
E Hypertension
F Immunosuppression
G Peptic ulcer disease
H Trigeminal neuralgia

For each of the following drugs that cause reactions in the gingivae, choose the most appropriate use from the list above. You may use each option once, more than once or not at all.

1 Phenytoin
2 Ciclosporin
3 Nifedipine
4 Sulphonamides
5 Methotrexate

6.15 Theme: Treatment Options and the BPE

A Nothing
B Oral hygiene instructions (OHI)
C OHI and scaling
D OHI, scaling and root debridement, consider gingival surgery
E Alter restoration
F OHI and deep scaling

For each of the following statements, choose the most appropriate treatment from the list above. You may use each option once, more than once or not at all.

1 One or more tooth in a sextant has a pocket of greater than 6 mm.
2 No pocketing, but an overhang is present on a restoration.
3 In a sextant there is pocketing of 4 or 5 mm but nothing greater.
4 There is gingivitis present but no pocketing.
5 The deepest pockets in the sextant are 2 mm.

6.16 Theme: Curettage

A All teeth
B All anterior teeth
C Distal surfaces of posterior teeth
D Mesial surfaces of posterior teeth
E Buccal and lingual surfaces of posterior teeth
F Horizontally
G Obliquely
H Vertically
I Vertically, horizontally and obliquely

For each of the following questions regarding Gracey curettes, choose the most appropriate option from the list above. You may use each option once, more than once or not at all.

1 Where would you scale using a Gracey number 2 curette?
2 Where would you scale using a Gracey number 7 or 8 curette?
3 Where would you scale using a Gracey number 13 or 14 curette?
4 Where would you scale using a Gracey number 15 or 16 curette?
5 In which direction should you move a Gracey curette when scaling?

6.17 Theme: Periodontal Probes

A 1 g
B 5 g
C 25 g
D 50 g
E 250 g
F 0.1 mm
G 0.5 mm
H 1 mm
I 1.5 mm
J Epidemiological screening
K Calculus detection
L Accurate pocket depth measurement
M To perform a basic periodontal examination (BPE)

For each of the following questions regarding periodontal probes, choose the most appropriate option from the list above. You may use each option once, more than once or not at all.

1 With a World Health Organization (WHO) probe what pressure should you be using when placing it into a pocket?
2 What is a WHO probe used for?
3 What is the size of the ball on the end of a WHO probe?
4 What is a CPITN-C probe used for?
5 What is a Williams probe used for?

6.18 Theme: Down Syndrome

A	1	K	Sex-linked
B	16	L	Non-disjunction
C	21	M	Habitual self-harm of the gingivae
D	27	N	Smoking
E	1:100	O	Macroglossia
F	1:400	P	Delayed eruption of the dentition
G	1:800	Q	Cyanotic heart disease
H	1:1500	R	Duodenal atresia
I	Autosomal recessive	S	Tracheo-oesophageal fistula
J	Autosomal dominant		

For each of the following questions, choose the most appropriate option from the list above. You may use each option once, more than once or not at all.

1. Which chromosome is affected in most cases?
2. What is the proportion of live births with Down syndrome?
3. How is Down syndrome inherited in the majority of cases?
4. Which local factor in Down syndrome causes worsening of periodontal disease?
5. Which congenital abnormality associated with Down syndrome may complicate treatment?

6.19 Theme: Gingivostomatitis

A	Aciclovir	H	4
B	Amoxicillin	I	5
C	Erythromycin	J	7
D	Tetracycline	K	10
E	1	L	14
F	2	M	21
G	3		

For each of the following questions regarding herpetic gingivostomatitis, choose the most appropriate option from the list above. You may use each option once, more than once or not at all.

1. What is the drug of choice?
2. How many times a day is this drug taken?
3. What age (years) does this usually present?
4. What is the number of the herpesvirus which causes this condition?
5. How long (days) does it last for?

PERIODONTICS

6.20 Theme: Gram Staining

A   Positive
B   Negative
C   Does not stain with Gram stain

For each of the following bacteria, choose the most appropriate option from the list above with regard to their Gram staining. You may use each option once, more than once or not at all.

1 Porphyromonas gingivalis
2 Prevotella intermedia
3 Actinobacillus actinomycetemcomitans
4 Treponema pallidum
5 Streptococcus mutans

6.21 Theme: Papillon–Lefèvre Disease

A   Autosomal dominant
B   Autosomal recessive
C   Sex-linked
D   1
E   11
F   20
G   31
H   41
I   1:1000
J   1:10 000
K   1:100 000
L   1:1 000 000
M   Male
N   Female
O   Equally distributed between males and females

For each of the following questions, choose the most appropriate option from the list above. You may use each option once, more than once or not at all.

1 How is Papillon–Lefèvre disease inherited?
2 Which chromosome is it associated with?
3 What is the age of onset?
4 What is the prevalence?
5 In which sex is it more prevalent?

6.22 Theme: Immunoglobulins

A   IgA
B   IgD
C   IgE
D   IgG
E   IgM

For each of the following statements, choose the most appropriate immunoglobulin from the list above. You may use each option once, more than once or not at all.

1 Most prevalent immunoglobulin.
2 It is a dimer.
3 It is a pentamer.
4 It is mainly found on the surface of B cells and found in the smallest amount.
5 Causes type 1 hypersensitivity and reacts with mast cells.

6.23 Theme: Diabetes

A   × 1
B   × 5
C   × 20
D   × 50
E   × 250
F   Type 1 diabetes
G   Type 2 diabetes
H   Thickens blood vessel lumen
I   Thins blood vessel lumen
J   Has no effect on blood vessel lumen
K   1.5–3.5 mmol/l
L   3.5–5.5 mmol/l
M   5.5–7.5 mmol/l
N   7.5–9.5 mmol/l

For each of the following questions, choose the most appropriate option from the list above. You may use each option once, more than once or not at all.

1 If you smoke, have diabetes and are over 45 years of age, what is your relative risk of getting periodontal disease?
2 Which type of diabetes has a family history?
3 Which type of diabetes does not have a family history?
4 What is the effect of diabetes on the lumen of blood vessels?
5 What is the normal fasting venous glucose value?

6.24 Theme: Topical Antimicrobials

A	Chlorhexidine gluconate
B	Clindamycin
C	Hyaluronic acid
D	Metronidazole
E	Minocycline

For each of the following common topical antimicrobials used in the treatment of periodontal disease, choose the most appropriate active ingredient from the list above. You may use each option once, more than once or not at all.

1. Gengigel
2. Dentomycin
3. PerioChip
4. Elyzol
5. Corsodyl

6.25 Theme: Indices

A	0
B	1
C	2
D	3
E	4
F	5
G	6
H	*
I	-

For each of the following statements relating to the indices in parenthesis, choose the most appropriate grade from the list above. You may use each option once, more than once or not at all.

1. Movement of a crown in the horizontal plane is greater than 1 mm (Tooth mobility index)
2. No teeth are present in a sextant (BPE)
3. A furcation lesion is present in a sextant (BPE)
4. Soft debris covering over two-thirds of the tooth (Debris index)
5. Movement of the crown in a vertical plane (Tooth mobility index)

6.26 Theme: Periodontal Instruments

A   Chisel
B   Curette
C   Hoe
D   Sickle

For each of the following instruments, choose the most appropriate name from the list above. You may use each option once, more than once or not at all.

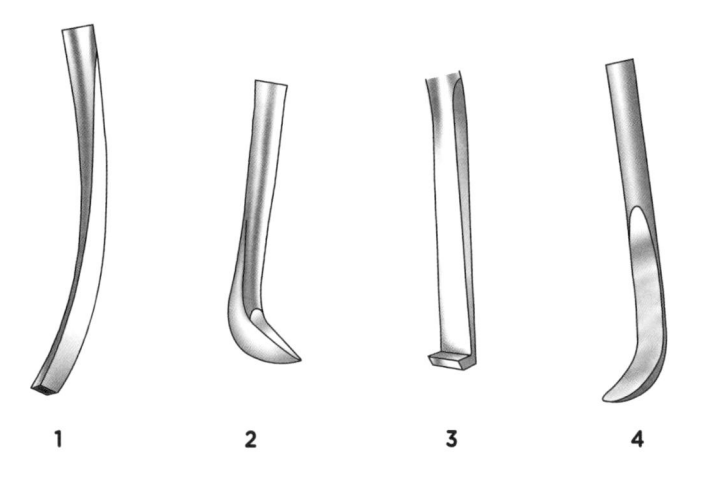

1

2

3

4

6.1 Syndromes associated with Gingival Overgrowth

1	D	Laband
2	D	Laband
3	C	Cross
4	E	Ramon
5	F	Rutherfurd

The following syndromes are not associated with gingival fibromatosis:

Apert syndrome. Cranio-facial syntosis with facial dysmorphology, limb defects and learning disability.

Chediak–Higashi syndrome. Congenital immune deficiency, early-onset aggressive periodontitis, early tooth loss and oral ulceration.

Turner syndrome. Affects females only, short stature, web neck, broad chest, occasionally cherubism.

6.2 Gracey Curettes

1	D	7/8
2	G	13/14
3	I	17/18
4	D	7/8
5	F	11/12

Curettes are either universal or site-specific, such as Gracey curettes. Curettes have a rounded toe, rounded back and are semi-circular in cross-section. Universal curettes are designed for easy adaption to all root surfaces, hence the name universal. Gracey curettes are site-specific with one cutting edge. 1/2, 3/4 are for incisor and canine root surfaces, 5/6 is also for anterior teeth and premolars. 7/8 is for buccal and lingual surfaces of premolars and molars. 9/10 is for buccal and lingual surfaces of molars. 11/12 for mesial surfaces of premolars and molars. 13/14 for distal surfaces of premolars and molars. The curette 15/16 is used for the removal of subgingival plaque, calculus and root-planing of the mesial surfaces in the premolar/molar areas. This is the same as the Gracey curette 11/12; however, the more accentuated angulation of the shank makes it easier to access the posterior areas; similarly, 17/18 is for root surface debridement of distal surfaces of premolars/molars like 13/14, but more accentuated angulation of the shank, making it particularly good for the distal surface of third molars.

6.3 Local Drug Delivery in the Management of Periodontal Diseases

1 E Minocycline

2 C Doxycycline

3 D Metronidazole

4 B Chlorhexidine

5 E Minocycline

Arestin has 1 mg of minocycline hydrochloride in polymer to allow sustained release in the gingival cervical fluid for up to 14 days.

Atridox is 10% by weight doxycycline hyclate in a polymer for controlled release for up to 7 days. Another brand using doxycycline as the active ingredient is Doxy.

Elyzol is 25% metronidazole benzoate in glyceryl mono-oleate and sesame oil.

PerioChip is 2.5 mg chlorhexidine gluconate in a gelatine matrix diffusing out over 7 days. Another brand using chlorhexidine as the active ingredient is Chlo-site.

Periocline is 2.1 % minocycline hydrochloride in a hydroxyethyl-cellulose matrix.

Azithromycin 0.5% is relatively new in the treatment of periodontal disease by local delivery and has been used in some studies.

6.4 Periodontitis as a Manifestation of Systemic Disease

1   D   Down syndrome

2   I   Papillon-Lefèvre syndrome

3   G   Histiocytosis

4   H   Hypophosphatasia

5   E   Ehlers-Danlos syndrome

Down syndrome is caused by trisomy of the chromosome 21. IQ is lowered, and there are characteristic facial features and periodontal disease especially affecting the incisor and molar teeth.

Papillon-Lefèvre syndrome is an uncommon autosomal recessive palmoplantar ectodermal dysplasia. Premature loss of teeth usually occurs.

Histiocytosis is a general name for a group of syndromes that involve an increase in histiocytes. Swelling looseness and tenderness of the teeth occur usually in childhood.

Hypophosphatasia is an inherited disorder with defected mineralisation of bone and teeth. Early loss of teeth usually occurs in childhood.

Ehlers-Danlos syndrome is characterised by collagen synthesis defects, hence the loose joints and periodontal disease.

Asperger syndrome is *not* associated with periodontal disease but is on the autistic spectrum.

Chediak-Higashi syndrome is associated with severe periodontal disease due to neutrophil abnormalities.

Cohen syndrome is autosomal-recessive and is characterised by mental and motor retardation, obesity, neutropenia and periodontal disease.

All neutropenias result in some form of periodontal disease.

6.5 Systemic Diseases associated with Periodontal Disease

1   A   Chediak-Higashi syndrome

2   C   Down syndrome

PERIODONTICS

3 G Histiocytosis syndrome

4 J Papillon-Lefèvre syndrome

Soft tissue lesions of the oral cavity are common in children, and distinguishing between findings that are normal and those that are indicative of gingivitis, periodontal disease, local or systemic infection, and potentially life-threatening systemic conditions is important. The loss of the periodontal attachment in children, manifested as tooth mobility or premature loss, can be a symptom of neoplasia, immunodeficiency or metabolic defects.

6.6 Micro-organisms

1 I *Streptococcus mutans*

2 K *Streptococcus sanguis*

3 E *Lactobacillus*

4 F *Porphyromonas gingivalis*

5 G *Treponema pallidum*

6 D *Candida albicans*

7 B *Actinomyces israelii*

8 A *Actinobacillus actinomycetemcomitans*

9 H *Streptococcus milleri*

10 C *Borrelia vincentii*

It is important to know about bacteria and their role in periodontal disease. In the different types of periodontal disease, different bacteria are implicated, and knowledge of these different situations is needed for finals.

6.7 Plaque, Pellicle, Gingivitis and Calculus

1 F Streptococci

2 G *Actinomyces*

3 J Gram-negative bacteria

4 I Gram-positive bacteria

5 D 80%

To ensure that you are able to differentiate between gingivitis and periodontal disease it is important to have knowledge about the histopathology of both conditions and a good knowledge of inflammation.

6.8 Risk Factors

1 C Epulis

2 B ANUG

3 A Acute bleeding

4 D Hyperplasia

5 E Periodontal disease of the deciduous dentition

Pregnancy causes hormonal disturbances leading to the formation of a pregnancy epulis, usually in an area associated with poor plaque control. The treatment of choice is good debridement of the area rather than excision of the epulis, as it can be extremely vascular. Smoking is a major factor in the development of ANUG in many patients. ANUG is associated with the characteristic fetor oris and widespread painful ulceration. Spontaneous frank bleeding of the gingivae should always be investigated, especially in patients with good oral hygiene. Leukaemia or other blood dyscrasias should always be ruled out. A patient who has had a renal transplant is likely to be taking ciclosporin, which has gingival hyperplasia as a side-effect. Chediak–Higashi disease is a rare autosomal recessive disorder affecting the function of neutrophils, and leads to the rapid loss of both deciduous and permanent dentition.

PERIODONTICS

6.9 Basic Periodontal Examination

1 E 4

2 C 2

3 D 3

4 C 2

5 B 1

The WHO probe is used to perform a basic periodontal examination. The scores are explained in the table below.

Score	Disease
0	No disease
1	Gingival bleeding, no overhangs or calculus, pockets < 3.5 mm
2	No pockets > 3.5 mm, no supragingival calculus or subgingival overhangs present
3	Pockets within the colour-coded area 3.5 mm to 5.5 mm
4	Colour-coded area disappears, pockets > 5.5 mm

6.10 ANUG

1 D   Africa

2 J   Cancrum oris

3 F   *Spirochaetes*

4 AA 25–40 years

5 O   Male

6	S	Punched out
7	V	Debridement, antibiotics and mouthwash
8	EE	Peroxyl
9	W	Metronidazole
10	L	AIDS

ANUG is predominantly found in males between the ages of 25 and 40 years. The predisposing factors are poor oral hygiene, smoking, systemic disease and poorly functioning immune system. The patient presents with a characteristic fetor oris and painful punched out ulceration of the interdental papillae covered by a pseudomembrane. The treatment of choice is debridement under local anaesthetic, complemented by metronidazole and a sodium perborate mouthwash. Chlorhexidine is not used because the pseudomembrane prevents its action. The sodium perborate is useful in this case.

6.11 Juvenile Periodontitis – Epidemiology

1	C	0.1%
2	B	0.05%
3	I	Black
4	K	Male
5	N	Good

6.12 Juvenile Periodontitis

1 B Molars

2 C Incisors

3 E *Actinomyces actinomycetemcomitans*

4 K Neutrophil chemotaxis

5 N Tetracycline

Juvenile periodontitis occurs mainly in males, and is 30 times more prevalent in the Black population. It has an overall prevalence of 0.6%. It initially presents with mobility of the molar teeth, followed by the incisors. It is thought that this is because of the order of eruption of the permanent teeth. Surprisingly patients with this condition tend to have good oral hygiene. It is caused by *Actinobacillus actinomycetemcomitans* and responds quite well to tetracycline. It does seem to have a genetic link, and patients seem to have a higher prevalence of neutrophil chemotaxis disorders.

6.13 Lateral Periodontal Abscess

1 A No pain

2 E Sensitive to lateral percussion

3 H Always pocketing

4 J Vital

5 L Vertical bone loss

Lateral periodontal abscesses are usually found in vital teeth where the tooth is sensitive to lateral percussion rather than apical percussion. There is usually evidence of a local vertical bony lesion on a radiograph, and clinically there is always pocketing.

6.14 Drugs and Periodontal Disease

1 D Epilepsy

2 F Immunosuppression

3 E Hypertension

4 B Antibiotic

5 C Chemotherapeutic drug

A medical and drug history is very important with all patients. This may explain unusual problems with gingivae. The classic question is regarding gingival hyperplasia, which can be caused by calcium-channel blockers, phenytoin and ciclosporin. Sulphonamides may cause desquamative gingivitis.

6.15 Treatment Options and the BPE

1 D OHI, scaling and root debridement, consider gingival surgery

2 E Alter restoration

3 F OHI and deep scaling

4 B OHI

5 C OHI and scaling

A finals student should be able to suggest a treatment plan for various situations. The questions above cover most of the simple periodontal scenarios. Getting these wrong does not give a good impression to the examiner.

PERIODONTICS

6.16 Curettage

1	B	All anterior teeth
2	E	Buccal and lingual surfaces of posterior teeth
3	C	Distal surfaces of posterior teeth
4	D	Mesial surfaces of posterior teeth
5	I	Vertically, horizontally and obliquely

It is important to recognise and know which instruments are used and where. A good tip is if you are unsure look at the instrument and it usually has its name written on it somewhere!

6.17 Periodontal Probes

1	C	25 g
2	J	Epidemiological screening
3	G	0.5 mm
4	M	To perform a BPE
5	L	Accurate pocket depth measurement

Students should know which probes to use and when to use them.

6.18 Down Syndrome

1	C	21
2	G	1:800
3	L	Non-disjunction
4	O	Macroglossia
5	Q	Cyanotic heart disease

Down syndrome is caused in the majority of cases by the non-disjunction of chromosome 21. It occurs in 1:800 of live births, but the prevalence increases with maternal age up to 1:100, if the mother is 40+ years of age. Down's children have delayed eruption of the dentition; however, this does not affect the periodontium. Because of macroglossia, Down's children tend to mouth breathe, which exacerbates their predisposition to periodontal disease. They also have a higher prevalence of congenital abnormalities of the heart, especially atrial septal defects and Fallot's tetralogy. These conditions require antibiotic prophylaxis if surgical correction has taken place.

6.19 Gingivostomatitis

1	A	Aciclovir
2	I	5
3	E	1
4	E	1
5	K	10

Primary herpetic gingivostomatitis usually occurs in children who are teething and lasts for up to 10 days. Only in severe cases is aciclovir required. Most children respond well to fluids and analgesia.

6.20 Gram Staining

1	B	Negative
2	B	Negative
3	B	Negative
4	B	Negative
5	A	Positive

Microbiology is a very important subset of periodontology. Knowing whether a bacterium is Gram positive or Gram negative enables you to work out how the bacterium is pathogenic.

6.21 Papillon-Lefèvre Disease

1	B	Autosomal recessive
2	E	11
3	D	1
4	L	1:1 000 000
5	O	Equally distributed between males and females

Papillon-Lefèvre causes early loss of the deciduous and permanent dentition. It is an autosomal recessive disorder associated with chromosome 11. It occurs equally in males and females. Other problems include superficial keratoses and plaques, neutrophil dysfunction, nail changes, bacterial susceptibility and liver abscesses.

6.22 Immunoglobulins

1 D IgG

2 A IgA

3 E IgM

4 B IgD

5 C IgE

A basic knowledge of immunology is important so that the student knows how to explain the body's reaction to bacteria.

6.23 Diabetes

1 C × 20

2 G Type 2 diabetes

3 F Type 1 diabetes

4 H Thickens blood vessel lumen

5 L 3.5–5.5 mmol/l

Diabetes mellitus is one of the major risk factors for periodontal disease. There are two major types: type 1 (insulin-dependent diabetes mellitus (IDDM)) and type 2 (non-insulin dependent diabetes mellitus (NIDDM)). Type 2 is familial and type 1 is non-familial. They both cause the thickening of the lumen of blood vessels and this is thought to contribute to periodontal disease as it decreases blood flow. It is important for diabetic people to achieve good control over their blood glucose or the long-term effects of diabetes become more prevalent.

PERIODONTICS

6.24 Topical Antimicrobials

1	C	Hyaluronic acid
2	E	Minocycline
3	A	Chlorhexidine gluconate
4	D	Metronidazole
5	A	Chlorhexidine gluconate

Topical antimicrobials are useful in the treatment of periodontal disease. Knowing the correct contents of each of the above topical antimicrobials is important.

6.25 Indices

1	C	2
2	I	-
3	H	*
4	D	3
5	D	3

Tooth mobility is graded as shown in the table below.

Grade	Description
1	Movement of the crown of a tooth in the horizontal plane is 0.2-1 mm
2	Movement of the crown of a tooth in the horizontal plane is > 1 mm
3	Movement of the crown of a tooth in the vertical plane

The Debris index is shown in the table below.

PERIODONTICS

ANSWERS

Grade	Description
0	No debris or stain
1	Soft debris or stain covering not more than one-third of the tooth surface
2	Soft debris or stain covering between one-third and two-thirds of the tooth surface
3	Soft debris or stain covering > two-thirds of the tooth surface

6.26 Periodontal Instruments

1 A Chisel

2 D Sickle

3 C Hoe

4 B Curette

It is important that final year students are able to recognise basic hand instruments.

7 Pharmacology

7.1 Theme: Drug Treatment for Hypertension
7.2 Theme: Drugs and Pregnancy (1)
7.3 Theme: Pain Control
7.4 Theme: Side-effects (1)
7.5 Theme: Vitamins
7.6 Theme: Side-effects (2)
7.7 Theme: Drugs and their Side-effects (1)
7.8 Theme: Drugs and their Side-effects (2)
7.9 Theme: Mechanisms of Action of Common Drugs
7.10 Theme: Hypoglycaemia
7.11 Theme: Blood Pressure and Ischaemic Heart Disease
7.12 Theme: Cardiovascular Emergencies
7.13 Theme: Diabetes
7.14 Theme: Antibiotics (1)
7.15 Theme: Adverse Drug Reactions
7.16 Theme: Acute Asthma and Chronic Obstructive Pulmonary Disease (COPD)
7.17 Theme: Practical Prescribing
7.18 Theme: Asthma and COPD
7.19 Theme: Overdose
7.20 Theme: Drug Interaction
7.21 Theme: Drugs and the Liver
7.22 Theme: Drugs and Misuse
7.23 Theme: Polypharmacy
7.24 Theme: Drugs and Pregnancy (2)
7.25 Theme: Statistical Terminology
7.26 Theme: Clinical Trials
7.27 Theme: Treatment of Arthritis
7.28 Theme: Common Arrhythmias
7.29 Theme: Antibiotics (2)

7.1 Theme: Drug Treatment for Hypertension

A ACE Inhibitors
B Alfa blockers
C Angiotensin II antagonists
D Beta blockers
E Calcium channel blockers
F Thiazide diuretics

For each of the descriptions below, choose the most appropriate treatment from the list above. Each option may be used once, more than once or not at all.

1. Also used to treat prostatism.
2. Avoid in patients with peripheral vascular disease.
3. Can cause profound hypotension.
4. Postural hypotension is a common side-effect.
5. May precipitate gout.
6. Sleep disturbances frequently reported.

7.2 Theme: Drugs and Pregnancy (1)

A Arthropathy
B Cranial nerve VIII damage
C General teratogenicity
D Hypoglycaemia
E Hypothyroidism
F No harmful effects reported
G Osteoporosis
H Tooth discoloration

For each of the following drugs, choose which effect on the fetus they make have from the list above. Each option may be used once, more than once or not at all.

1. Aminoglycosides
2. Cefotaxine
3. Fluconazole
4. Heparin
5. Tetracycline
6. Trimethoprim

7.3 Theme: Pain Control

A   Amitriptyline
B   Aspirin
C   Co-dydramol
D   Diamorphine
E   Diclofenac
F   Fentanyl
G   Paracetamol

For each of the following scenarios, choose the most appropriate drug from the list below. Each option may be used once, more than once or not at all.

1. A 10-year-old female with irreversible pulpitis.
2. A 2-year-old male with a dry socket.
3. A 45-year-old female with post-herpetic neuralgia.
4. A 52-year-old male with a renal calculus.
5. A 80-year-old male with acute myocardial infarction.

7.4 Theme: Side-effects (1)

A   Anorgasmia
B   Convulsions
C   Gingival hyperplasia
D   Haemorrhagic cystitis
E   Jaundice
F   Neutropenia
G   Osteopenia
H   Peripheral neuropathy

For each of the following drugs, choose the most characteristic side-effect from the list below. Each option may be used once, more than once or not at all.

1. Carbimazole
2. Clozapine
3. Corticosteroids
4. Isoniazid
5. Lignocaine
6. Phenytoin

7.5 Theme: Vitamins

A	Vitamin A	E	Vitamin C
B	Vitamin B_1	F	Vitamin D
C	Vitamin B_6	G	Vitamin E
D	Vitamin B_{12}	H	Vitamin K

For each of the following statements, choose the most appropriate vitamin supplement from the list below. Each option may be used once, more than once or not at all.

1. Asian women and house bound elderly may need supplementation.
2. Hypercalcaemia may occur with high doses.
3. Treatment for pernicious anaemia.
4. Self-supplementation contraindicated in pregnancy.
5. Used to prevent Wernicke's encephalopathy.
6. Used to treat scurvy.

7.6 Theme: Side-effects (2)

A	Acute confusion	F	Head injury
B	Alcohol dependency	G	Hypoglycaemia
C	Alzheimer's disease	H	Meningitis
D	Depression	I	Parkinson's disease
E	Drug overdose	J	Psychotic episode

For each of the following scenarios, select the best primary diagnosis from the list above. You may use each option once, more than once or not at all.

1. An elderly woman attending for her appointment seems more confused than you recall on the last visit. She is not taking any medications. Her daughter, who is accompanying her, says she has seemed vague for the past 2 days and is complaining of burning when she passes urine.

2. A 55-year-old man is noted to have bruises on his arms and legs and smells of alcohol. On sensitive questioning, he admits to not being able to start the day without having four glasses of whisky and has lost his job after being drunk at work recently.

3. An elderly woman attending for fitting of her dentures tells you she is worried that her memory has deteriorated over the past 6 months and she keeps forgetting where she has left her purse and keys. She has not had any falls and denies any tremor in her hands.

PHARMACOLOGY

7.7 Theme: Drugs and their Side-effects (1)

A	Atorvastatin	F	Methotrexate
B	Co-amoxiclav	G	Metoprolol
C	Doxycycline	H	Paracetamol
D	Furosemide	I	Thyroxine
E	Ibuprofen	J	Warfarin

For each of the following scenarios, select the most likely responsible agent from the list above. You may use each option once, more than once or not at all.

1. An 85-year-old man was given antibiotics for a dental abscess and has now developed yellowish, offensive diarrhoea.

2. A 56-year-old man complains of central burning chest pain after eating a big meal. This occurs most evenings after dinner and is often relieved by taking an antacid. He denies any previous heart disease but takes pain relief for his osteoarthritis.

3. A 67-year-old man who recently had a myocardial infarction has noticed that he sometimes feels dizzy and faint. When you take his pulse, it is 45 bpm.

7.8 Theme: Drugs and their Side-effects (2)

A	Acarbose
B	Ciprofloxacin
C	Codeine phosphate
D	Diclofenac
E	Erythromycin
F	Glibenclamide
G	Orlistat
H	Paracetamol
I	Primrose oil
J	Sibutramine

For each of the following side-effects, select the most likely responsible medication from the list above. You may use each option once, more than once or not at all.

1. Diarrhoea, intestinal cramping and involuntary leakage of fatty stools.
2. Constipation.
3. Episodes of hypoglycaemia, if not taken with food.

7.9 Theme: Mechanisms of Action of Common Drugs

A	Anti-cholinesterase inhibitor
B	Blocks the Na/K transporter in the loop of Henle
C	Bronchoconstrictor
D	Chain-terminating antiviral
E	Cyclo-oxygenase (COX) (enzyme) inhibitor
F	Decreases seizure threshold
G	Inhibits coagulation factors II, V, VII and IX
H	Prevents reabsorption of bile salts
I	Peripheral vasodilator
J	Smooth-muscle relaxant

For each of the following drugs choose the most appropriate mechanism of action in the list above. You may use each option once, more than once or not at all.

1. Isosorbide mononitrate.
2. Furosemide.
3. Aspirin.

7.10 Theme: Hypoglycaemia

A	0.9% saline and short-acting intravenous insulin
B	0.9% saline, short-acting intravenous insulin and potassium
C	50% glucose and short-acting insulin
D	50 ml of 5% glucose intravenously
E	50 ml of 50% glucose intravenously
F	Acarbose
G	Gliclazide
H	Heparin
I	Metformin
J	Oral glucose solution
K	Short-acting insulin

For each of the following scenarios, choose the most appropriate treatment option from the list above. You may use each option once, more than once or not at all.

1. A conscious 18-year-old man with type 1 diabetes presents in the dental surgery with sweating, anxiety and tachycardia due to hypoglycaemia.

2. A 64-year-old man with type 2 diabetes and raised blood glucose and sodium levels is already being treated with intravenous insulin and saline. What drug should be added?

3. A 24-year-old man with type 1 diabetes is brought to accident and emergency (A&E) comatose, with a blood glucose of 1.5 mmol/l. What is the correct treatment?

4. A 70-year-old man taking only metformin, presents with high blood glucose and high HbA1c levels. Which drug should be added to his regimen?

5. A 30-year-old man presents with type 1 diabetes and metabolic acidosis, and raised glucose and raised potassium levels. What is the correct treatment?

7.11 Theme: Blood Pressure and Ischaemic Heart Disease

- A   Adenosine
- B   Atenolol
- C   Atropine
- D   Clopidogrel
- E   Enalapril
- F   Furosemide
- G   Indometacin
- H   Intravenous low-molecular-weight heparin
- I   Low-dose aspirin
- J   Streptokinase
- K   Subcutaneous low-molecular-weight heparin
- L   Sublingual glyceryl trinitrate

For each of the following scenarios, choose the most appropriate treatment option from the list above. You may use each option once, more than once or not at all.

1. Antiplatelet therapy for a patient with known atherosclerosis.
2. Immediate relief of exertional angina.
3. Treatment of hypertension in a 70-year-old man with angina.
4. Thrombolysis for a 50-year-old man having an acute myocardial infarction.
5. Anticoagulation for a patient with unstable angina.

7.12 Theme: Cardiovascular Emergencies

- A Aspirin
- B Aspirin, atenolol
- C Aspirin, atenolol and streptokinase
- D Aspirin, heparin and glyceryl trinitrate
- E Aspirin and streptokinase
- F Intravenous glyceryl trinitrate
- G Low-molecular-weight heparin
- H Low-molecular-weight heparin and atenolol
- I Oral atenolol
- J Oral glyceryl trinitrate
- K Sublingual nifedipine

For each of the following scenarios, choose the most appropriate drug(s) from the list above. You may use each option once, more than once or not at all.

1. A 70-year-old man with asthma and a 10-minute history of chest pain, whose ECG shows ST depression, indicative of ischaemia.

2. A 55-year-old man with acute pulmonary oedema and a blood pressure of 160/105 mmHg.

3. A 55-year-old man with a 3-hour history of severe chest pain and ECG changes indicative of an acute myocardial infarction and bradycardia.

4. A 45-year-old man with blood pressure of 240/140 mmHg, grade IV retinopathy and proteinuria.

5. A 60-year-old woman with an acute thrombotic stroke.

7.13 Theme: Diabetes

A	Chlorphenamine
B	Furosemide
C	Glibenclamide
D	Glucagon
E	Long-acting insulin
F	Losartan
G	Low-calorie diabetic diet with low-sodium diet and exercise
H	Low-dose aspirin
I	Metformin
J	Rosiglitazone
K	Short-acting insulin
L	Spironolactone

For each of the following scenarios, choose the most appropriate treatment option from the list above. You may use each option once, more than once or not at all.

1. Alternative hypoglycaemic treatment for a 60-year-old man with poorly controlled blood glucose, despite maximum doses of oral hypoglycaemic drugs.

2. A 57-year-old obese man with type 2 diabetes has poorly controlled blood glucose. He is not taking any medication.

3. A 45-year-old man with type 2 diabetes has symptoms of hyperglycaemia. However, he has chronic renal failure.

4. A 75-year-old woman with type 2 diabetes requiring control of perioperative blood glucose levels.

5. A 40-year-old overweight male with mild type 2 diabetes and mild hypertension. He is not taking any medication.

7.14 Theme: Antibiotics (1)

A   Amoxicillin and flucloxacillin
B   Cefotaxime
C   Clarithromycin
D   Erythromycin and amoxicillin
E   Flucloxacillin and fusidic acid
F   Intravenous cefuroxime
G   Intravenous erythromycin
H   Oral gentamicin
I   Oral nitrofurantoin
J   Rifampicin
K   Tetracycline

For each of the following scenarios, choose the most appropriate treatment option from the list above. You may use each option once, more than once or not at all.

1   Outpatient prophylaxis for recurrent urinary tract infection in a 30-year-old woman.

2   Treatment of osteomyelitis caused by *Staphylococcus aureus* in a 40-year-old intravenous drug misuser.

3   Initial treatment of a 22-year-old woman with fever, rigors and abdominal pain caused by acute pyelonephritis.

4   Initial treatment of a 67-year-old man with community-acquired lobar pneumonia.

5   Initial treatment of meningitis in a teenager.

7.15 Theme: Adverse Drug Reactions

A	Diamorphine
B	Digoxin
C	Doxazosin
D	Ibuprofen
E	Intravenous adenosine
F	Lignocaine
G	Low-dose aspirin
H	Simvastatin
I	Verapamil
J	Warfarin

For each of the following scenarios, choose the most appropriate option from the list above. You may use each option once, more than once or not at all.

1. A 46-year-old man with muscle aches and pains 3 months after a myocardial infarction, taking drugs for secondary prevention.

2. Two weeks after starting treatment for atrial fibrillation, a 75-year-old man complains of nausea, constipation, abdominal discomfort and disturbed vision.

3. A 65-year-old woman on monotherapy for hypertension presents with constipation and ankle swelling.

4. A 60-year-old man presents with unsteadiness and falls. His blood pressure shows a postural drop.

5. A 50-year-old man with atrial fibrillation and nose bleeds.

7.16 Theme: Acute Asthma and Chronic Obstructive Pulmonary Disease (COPD)

A   Bolus of intravenous aminophylline
B   Broad-spectrum antibiotics, nebulised salbutamol, ipratropium bromide, oral prednisolone and 28% oxygen
C   Intravenous chlorphenamine, intramuscular adrenaline and intravenous hydrocortisone
D   Home oxygen
E   Nebulised ipratropium bromide
F   Nebulised salbutamol and ipratropium bromide, 60% oxygen, intravenous hydrocortisone and intravenous aminophylline
G   Nebulised salbutamol and 28% oxygen
H   Nebulised salbutamol, 60% oxygen and oral montelukast
I   Nebulised salbutamol, 60% oxygen, inhaled sodium cromoglycate
J   Nebulised salbutamol, 40% oxygen and prednisolone
K   40% oxygen, nebulised salbutamol and oral prednisolone
L   Salbutamol infusion

For each of the following scenarios, choose the most appropriate treatment option from the list above. You may use each option once, more than once or not at all.

1   Initial therapy for a 30-year-old man with life-threatening asthma.
2   Acute hypertension and wheeze following an acute anaphylactic reaction to penicillin.
3   A 30-year-old woman with acute severe asthma who is 20 weeks pregnant.
4   Add-on treatment for a 40-year-old man who has not responded to initial treatment for acute severe asthma. He is taking oral aminophylline.
5   A 74-year-old smoker with acute COPD.

7.17 Theme: Practical Prescribing

A   Case history sheet
B   Discharge medication sheet
C   Inpatient prescription chart – as required medication
D   Inpatient prescription chart – drugs with variable dosing schedules
E   Inpatient prescription chart – intravenous drugs with drug additives
F   Inpatient prescription chart – once-only medication
G   Inpatient prescription chart – regular medication
H   Nursing cardex
I   Patient observation chart
J   Surgical appliance request form

For each of treatments in the following scenarios, from the list above choose the most appropriate place where you would find them on a chart/form/sheet. You may use each option once, more than once or not at all.

1   Graduated compression hosiery for chronic venous insufficiency in a 90-year-old man with a post-phlebitic leg.

2   Diazepam as a pre-medication for a 45-year-old man undergoing repair of an inguinal hernia.

3   Chlordiazepoxide for a 55-year-old alcoholic with a fractured ankle at risk of alcohol withdrawal.

4   Bendrofluazide for long-standing hypertension in a 65-year-old man with cellulitis.

5   Soluble insulin for treatment of diabetic ketoacidosis in a 25-year-old man with type 1 diabetes.

7.18 Theme: Asthma and COPD

A   Home oxygen
B   Inhaled beclometasone
C   Inhaled ipratropium bromide
D   Inhaled salmeterol
E   Inhaled sodium cromoglycate
F   Oral diazepam
G   Oral ipratropium bromide
H   Oral montelukast
I   Oral prednisolone
J   Oral salbutamol
K   Oral theophylline
L   Salbutamol via metered-dose inhaler

For each of the following scenarios, choose the most appropriate add-on treatment option from the list above. You may use each option once, more than once or not at all.

1. Add-on treatment for a 20-year-old with asthma requiring daily administration of an inhaled β_2-agonist.

2. Add-on treatment for a 60-year-old smoker with dyspnoea secondary to COPD, despite inhalation treatment with a β_2-agonist and anticholinergic medication.

3. Add-on treatment for a 65-year-old smoker with persistent wheeze, despite inhaled β_2-agonist. He has good inhaler technique.

4. A 20-year-old woman with occasional symptoms of early morning wheeze caused by asthma.

5. Add-on treatment for a 25-year-old with asthma with persistent symptoms, despite treatment with a β_2-agonist and an inhaled steroid.

7.19 Theme: Overdose

A Acid diuresis
B Activated charcoal only
C Alkaline diuresis
D Atenolol intravenously
E Atropine intravenously
F Flumazenil intravenously
G Gastric lavage
H Induced emesis
I Methionine only
J Naloxone
K *N*-acetylcysteine intravenously
L Phosphate enema
M Salbutamol intravenously
N Vitamin K

For each of the following scenarios, choose the most appropriate treatment option from the list above. You may use each option once, more than once or not at all.

1. Treatment to decrease drug absorption in an 80-year-old woman who is depressed and reports she has swallowed 60 sleeping tablets.
2. Treatment for reversal of respiratory depression due to midazolam following extraction of wisdom teeth.
3. Salivation, bronchociliary secretion, miosis and abdominal pain in a soldier exposed to sarin nerve agent.
4. Respiratory depression in an 18-year-old intravenous drug misuser.
5. Paracetamol overdose in a dejected teenager with drug levels above the treatment line, 6 hours following ingestion.

7.20 Theme: Drug Interaction

A Confusion
B Constipation
C Postural hypotension
D Diarrhoea
E Dyspnoea and wheeze
F Hypertension
G Hypercalcaemia
H Neutropenia
I Taste disturbance
J Urinary obstruction

For each of the following scenarios, choose the most appropriate side-effect from the list above. You may use each option once, more than once or not at all.

1 A 73-year-old man taking fluoxetine for depression, and now taking misoprostol and diclofenac for arthritis.

2 A 55-year-old woman taking inhaled salbutamol for asthma, now prescribed timolol eye drops for glaucoma.

3 A 70-year-old man taking bendrofluazide and enalapril, started on doxazosin.

4 A 23-year-old woman with Hodgkin's lymphoma, being treated with vincristine and cyclophosphamide.

5 A 50-year-old treated with oxybutynin for bladder over-activity and dihydrocodeine for pain.

7.21 Theme: Drugs and the Liver

A	Alcohol	F	Methotrexate
B	Aspirin	G	Rifampicin
C	Codeine phosphate	H	Simvastatin
D	Folic acid	I	Spironolactone
E	Ibuprofen	J	Vitamin B$_1$

For each of the following hepatic complication scenarios, choose the most appropriate cause (drug) from the list above. You may use each option once, more than once or not at all.

1. Hepatic fibrosis in a 50-year-old woman with rheumatoid arthritis.
2. Right upper quadrant pain, jaundice, raised liver enzymes and coagulopathy in a 40-year-old publican.
3. Asymptomatic raised alanine aminotransferase in a 50-year-old man recovering from a myocardial infarction, on oral therapy for secondary prevention.
4. Coma in a constipated patient admitted with decompensated liver failure.
5. Unexpected pregnancy in a 26-year-old woman with tuberculosis.

7.22 Theme: Drugs and Misuse

A	Alcohol
B	Cannabis
C	Crack cocaine
D	Flunitrazepam (Rohypnol)
E	Heroin
F	Ketamine
G	LSD
H	MDMA (ecstasy)
I	Psilocybin (magic mushroom extract)

For each of the following descriptions, choose the most appropriate drug from the list above. You may use each option once, more than once or not at all.

1. A free base drug creating intense cramps on withdrawal.
2. Hallucinogenic drug with risk of flashback.
3. Sedative and mild hallucinogenic drug associated with chronic demotivational syndrome.
4. Hallucinogen used as a dissociative anaesthetic.
5. Opioid sedative, smoked or injected.

7.23 Theme: Polypharmacy

A	Aciclovir
B	Cholestyramine
C	Doxazosin
D	Erythromycin
E	Metolazone
F	Paracetamol
G	Prednisolone
H	Rifampicin
I	Spironolactone
J	Verapamil

In each of the following scenarios, the adverse event has been precipitated by a drug interaction between one of the drugs in the list above and the existing medication. For each scenario choose the most appropriate drug from the list above. You may use each option once, more than once or not at all.

1. Complete heart block in an 80-year-old man with hypertension and atrial fibrillation. He is treated with atenolol, digoxin, aspirin and bendrofluazide.

2. Profound hypokalaemia (K+ 2.0 mmol/l) in a 75-year-old man with heart failure and atrial fibrillation taking digoxin, warfarin and furosemide.

3. Hyperkalaemia (K+ 7.0 mmol/l) in a 70-year-old woman with heart failure and renal impairment already taking enalapril, hydrochlorothiazide/amiloride and aspirin.

4. Hyperglycaemia in a patient with type 2 diabetes following a controlled diet.

5. An international normalised ratio (INR) of 6 with nose bleeds in a 75-year-old man taking warfarin, digoxin and furosemide.

7.24 Theme: Drugs and Pregnancy (2)

A Aspirin
B Azithromycin
C Carbimazole
D Cefuroxime
E Chlorphenamine
F Enalapril
G Erythromycin
H Gentamicin
I Losartan
J Low-molecular-weight heparin
K Methyldopa
L Phenytoin
M Radioactive iodine
N Warfarin

For each of the following scenarios, choose the most appropriate treatment option from the list above. You may use each option once, more than once or not at all.

1. Hayfever in a 28-year-old woman who is 30 weeks pregnant.
2. Treatment of pulmonary embolism in a woman who is in her third trimester of pregnancy.
3. Acute pyelonephritis in a 24-year-old woman whose period is 2 weeks overdue.
4. Thyrotoxicosis in a pregnant woman.
5. Hypertension in a 40-year-old woman who is 23 weeks pregnant.

7.25 Theme: Statistical Terminology

A   Confidence interval
B   Mean
C   Median
D   Negative predictive value
E   Number needed to treat
F   Positive predictive value
G   Range
H   Sensitivity
I   Specificity
J   Standard deviation

For each of the following descriptions, choose the most appropriate term from the list above. You may use each option once, more than once or not at all.

1. A measure of the likelihood that a positive result means a patient has the disease.

2. (Number of disease-free people negative for the test/number of disease-free people) × 100.

3. A measure of the limits above and below mean value for a study population within which the true mean for the population lies.

4. Number of patients who would have to take a particular drug in order for one patient to benefit from taking it.

5. (Number of diseased people positive for a test/number of diseased people) × 100.

7.26 Theme: Clinical Trials

A   Absolute risk reduction
B   Bias
C   Confounding factors
D   Double blind
E   Number needed to treat
F   Open label
G   Real end point
H   Relative risk reduction
I   Single blind
J   Statistical power
K   Subgroup analysis
L   Surrogate end point

For each of the following descriptions, choose the most appropriate term from the list above. You may use each option once, more than once or not at all.

1 Re-analysis of trial to determine if treatment affects males more than females.

2 A clinical trial in which neither investigator nor patient is aware of the treatment allocation.

3 Stroke – in a trial investigating the effect of an antihypertensive drug on the cerebrovascular system.

4 Suppression of ventricular ectopic beats – in a trial to evaluate the function of anti-arrhythmic drugs after myocardial infarction.

5 In a clinical trial investigating a treatment for myocardial infarction, the percentage of patients with infarcts in the placebo group minus the percentage of patients with infarcts in the treatment group.

7.27 Theme: Treatment of Arthritis

A Allopurinol
B Aspirin
C Celecoxib
D Colchicine
E Diclofenac
F Ibuprofen and ranitidine
G Indometacin
H Infliximab
I Methotrexate and folic acid
J Paracetamol
K Prednisolone

For each of the following scenarios, choose the most appropriate treatment option from the list above. You may use each option once, more than once or not at all.

1. Reduction of inflammatory joint damage in a 65-year-old woman with severe rheumatoid arthritis who had previously received three disease-modifying antirheumatic drugs.

2. A 65-year-old man with recent history of gastric ulceration. His pain is not controlled by paracetamol and he requires a non-steroidal anti-inflammatory drug (NSAID) to control symptoms of rheumatoid arthritis.

3. Decrease in progressive joint damage in a 50-year-old woman with recently diagnosed rheumatoid arthritis.

4. Acute attack of gout in a 55-year-old man.

5. Treatment of muscle pain and stiffness in a 60-year-old man with polymyalgia rheumatica. His erythrocyte sedimentation rate (ESR) is markedly raised.

7.28 Theme: Common Arrhythmias

A　Adenosine
B　Aspirin
C　Clopidogrel
D　DC cardioversion
E　Intravenous amiodarone
F　Oral amiodarone
G　Verapamil
H　Warfarin for 4 weeks
I　Warfarin for life

For each of the following scenarios, choose the most appropriate option from the list above. You may use each option once, more than once or not at all.

1. Prophylaxis of atrio-ventricular nodal re-entry tachycardia in a 30-year-old asthmatic patient.

2. Maintenance of sinus rhythm in an 80-year-old man with a history of persistent atrial fibrillation that needs regular DC cardioversion.

3. Thromboembolic prophylaxis in an otherwise well 70-year-old man who has permanent atrial fibrillation and a history of thromboembolic stroke.

4. Restoration of sinus rhythm in a 70-year-old man who has become unwell on developing ventricular tachycardia.

5. Thromboembolic prophylaxis of a 50-year-old man, following a single episode of DC cardioversion for atrial fibrillation.

7.29 Theme: Antibiotics (2)

A	Amoxicillin
B	Cephaloridine
C	Clindamycin
D	Erythromycin
E	Flucloxacillin
F	Gentamicin
H	Metronidazole

For each of the following scenarios, choose the most appropriate treatment option from the list above. You may use each option once, more than once or not at all.

1. A 30-year-old patient attends for extraction of a tooth. There is a history of rheumatic fever, and they have not been prescribed antibiotics in the past 6 months and have no allergies.

2. A 56-year-old patient with a past history of rheumatic fever requires extractions. He had antibiotics the previous week to treat a dental abscess.

3. A 26-year-old woman presents with pericoronitis associated with submandibular lymphadenopathy and pyrexia. She has no relevant medical history.

4. A 20-year-old patient is diagnosed as having septicaemia with a positive blood culture, predominantly *Streptococcus milleri*. This is associated with carious lesions.

5. A 30-year-old woman presents with recurrent pain of the left maxillary region in the premolar area which is worse on bending down. It is associated with tenderness of the upper premolars and nasal discharge.

7.1 Drug Treatment for Hypertension

1 B Alfa blockers

2 D Beta blockers

3 A ACE Inhibitors

4 B Alfa blockers

5 F Thiazide diuretics

6 D Beta blockers

Prostatism is usually treated first with medicines called α blockers, such as doxazosin or terazosin. These drugs were first used to treat high blood pressure. Tamsulosin is the first alpha blocker developed specifically for benign prostate hyperplasia. These drugs relax the muscle in the prostate and at the bladder neck, which allows better urine flow.

Aggravation of intermittent claudication has been claimed to be a side-effect of β-blockade; however some research shows that β-blockers have little effect on peripheral circulation.

ACE-inhibitor-related hypotension is much more common in the setting of heart failure with reduced systolic function.

Alfa blockers, by reducing $α_1$-adrenergic activity of the blood vessels, may cause hypotension (low blood pressure) and interrupt the baroreflex response.

Hyperuricemia is a relatively common finding in patients treated with a loop or thiazide diuretic and may, over a period of time, lead to gouty arthritis.

Beta blockers are prescribed for cardiovascular disorders and anxiety. Many of the patients report having trouble sleeping, a side-effect possibly related to the fact that these medications suppress night-time melatonin production.

7.2 Drugs and Pregnancy (1)

1 B Cranial nerve VIII damage

2 F No harmful effects reported

3 C General teratogenicity

4 G Osteoporosis

5 H Tooth discoloration

6 C General teratogenicity

Hypoglycaemia may be caused by a large number of drugs namely Bactrim (an antibiotic), β-blockers, haloperidol, insulin, monoamine oxidase (MAO) inhibitors and metformin, when used with sulfonylureas, pentamidine and quinidine.

Hypothyroidism can be induced by a wide variety of drugs such as propylthiouracil (PTU), radioactive iodine, potassium iodide, and methimazole – also lithium or iodides in certain people. Unusual causes of drug-induced hypothyroidism include: amiodarone, eating a large amount of iodine-containing seaweed, nitroprusside, perchlorate, povidone iodine (Betadine) and sulfonylureas.

7.3 Pain Control

1 G Paracetamol

2 C Co-dydramol

3 A Amitriptyline

4 E Diclofenac

5 D Diamorphine

Paracetamol, also known as acetaminophen or APAP, is a widely used over-the-counter pain medication and antipyretic. It is commonly used for the relief of headaches and other minor aches and pains and is a major ingredient in numerous cold and flu remedies. Children should not be prescribed aspirin due to risk of Reye syndrome.

Co-dydramol tablets are used for the relief of moderate pain. Dry socket can be very painful and local measures such as dressing the socket will help to reduce the pain.

Post-herpetic neuralgia is a nerve pain due to damage caused by the varicella zoster virus. Typically, the neuralgia is confined to a dermatomic area of the skin and follows an outbreak of herpes zoster (shingles).

Low dosages of tricyclic antidepressants, including amitriptyline, seem to work best for deep, aching pain. These drugs affect key brain chemicals, including serotonin and norepinephrine, that play a role in both depression and how the body interprets pain. Doctors typically prescribe antidepressants for post-herpetic neuralgia in smaller doses than they do for depression.

Intramuscular diclofenac as a single agent for the treatment of renal colic is usually more effective than intramuscular tramadol. Intramuscular tramadol may be an alternative when contraindications preclude the use of diclofenac.

Diamorphine is an opiate, a type of drug extracted from the unripe seed capsules of the Asian poppy. It belongs to a group of drugs called the narcotic analgesics. The drug relieves the severe pain that can be caused by injury, surgery, myocardial infarction or chronic diseases such as cancer.

Intravenous fentanyl is often used for anaesthesia and analgesia. Fentanyl transdermal patch is used in chronic pain management.

7.4 Side-effects (1)

1 F Neutropenia

2 F Neutropenia

3 G Osteopenia

4 H Peripheral neuropathy

5 B Convulsions

6 C Gingival hyperplasia

Anorgasmia, or Coughlan's syndrome, is a type of sexual dysfunction in which a person cannot achieve orgasm despite adequate stimulation. The use of antidepressants, particularly selective serotonin reuptake inhibitors (SSRIs), may cause this as a side-effect.

Lignocaine has a concentration-dependent effect on convulsion/seizures.

Cyclophosphamide and anticancer chemotherapy or radiotherapy can cause haemorrhagic cystitis.

Jaundice can be a side-effect of many drugs.

Prolonged use of glucocorticoids can cause osteopenia.

7.5 Vitamins

1 F Vitamin D

2 F Vitamin D

3 D Vitamin B$_{12}$

4 A Vitamin A

5 B Vitamin B$_1$

6 E Vitamin C

Vitamin D requires exposure to sunlight, hence house-bound individuals frequently have low levels. Vitamins A, D, E and K are fat-soluble, and individuals on low-fat diets may develop deficiency. Vitamins B and C are water-soluble. Vitamin B is found in unprocessed vegetable sources, and vitamin C is found in fruits and vegetables.

7.6 Side-effects (2)

1 A Acute confusion

Elderly patients are prone to episodes of acute confusion, often precipitated by urine or chest infections. The history is too short to be due to a chronic dementing illness. There are no medications being taken that could cause low blood sugar.

2 B Alcohol dependency

This man may have had recurrent falls due to his alcohol problem but he does not display any features of a head injury in this scenario. He may well be concurrently depressed but the best answer to this stem is alcohol dependency.

3 C Alzheimer's disease

Alzheimer's is the commonest cause of chronic confusion in the elderly and often presents insidiously with short-term memory loss. Parkinson's disease is associated more with resting tremor and slowness of movement. It can cause chronic confusion but the woman does not have any symptoms to suggest this as the cause. She is unlikely to have a head injury, as there have been no recent falls.

PHARMACOLOGY

7.7 Drugs and their Side-effects (1)

1   B   Co-amoxiclav

Most antibiotics are associated with the risk of a *Clostridium difficile* infection. There are two antibiotics to choose from here. Doxycycline has less potential to promote *C. difficile* infection and is also not usually used to treat dental abscesses.

2   E   Ibuprofen

This man has indigestion, which can mimic cardiac chest pain. The fact that it is relieved by an antacid is reassuring, and the most likely culprit is an NSAID, eg ibuprofen. Paracetamol is another good painkiller used in osteoarthritis but it would not cause indigestion.

3   G   Metoprolol

After a myocardial infarction, patients are usually on β-blockers and statin tablets to reduce their cardiovascular risk. This man has a bradycardia, which is a common side-effect of β-blockers. Thyroxine in high doses is known to cause tachycardia.

7.8 Drugs and their Side-effects (2)

1   G   Orlistat

This is a weight-reducing drug approved by the National Institute for Health and Clinical Excellence (NICE), which acts by preventing the absorption of dietary fats. Hence, the symptoms of fatty stools and abdominal discomfort are common.

2   C   Codeine phosphate

This commonly used medication is an effective analgesic but can cause constipation if used for a prolonged time, particularly in elderly patients. Patients should be advised to drink plenty of water and see their GP if the problem persists.

3   F   Glibenclamide

This is a sulphonylurea which acts by increasing insulin secretion from the pancreas and is used in type 2 diabetes. If the tablets are taken without sufficient food intake, blood sugar levels may drop.

7.9 Mechanisms of Action of Common Drugs

1 I Peripheral vasodilator

This decreases total peripheral resistance and is used in heart failure and ischaemic heart disease. It may cause low blood pressure and headache when given.

2 B Blocks the Na/K transporter in the loop of Henle

This is a loop diuretic that acts by preventing sodium reabsorption in the nephron. Therefore, salt is excreted, along with water, hence its reputation as a 'water tablet'.

3 E COX (enzyme) inhibitor

NSAIDs, including aspirin, prevent platelet action by inhibiting the COX enzyme, thus preventing aggregation of platelets and reducing the risk of thrombus formation in vessels.

7.10 Hypoglycaemia

1 J Oral glucose solution

2 H Heparin

3 E 50 ml of 50% glucose intravenously

4 G Gliclazide

5 A 0.9% saline and short-acting intravenous insulin

In a dental surgery, the correct initial treatment for a patient who is having a hypoglycaemic episode is oral glucose solution. Heparin is an important drug for patients who have diabetic ketoacidosis, as they are likely to be dehydrated and the heparin will prevent any clotting episodes. HbA1c is a marker of the long-term effectiveness of diabetic control. It is low in patients with well-controlled diabetes.

PHARMACOLOGY

7.11 Blood Pressure and Ischaemic Heart Disease

1 I Low-dose aspirin

2 L Sublingual glyceryl trinitrate

3 B Atenolol

4 J Streptokinase

5 K Subcutaneous low-molecular-weight heparin

These are common treatments and must be known inside out!

7.12 Cardiovascular Emergencies

1 D Aspirin, heparin and glyceryl trinitrate

2 F Intravenous glyceryl trinitrate

3 E Aspirin and streptokinase

4 I Oral atenolol

5 A Aspirin

Intravenous glyceryl trinitrate is useful in pulmonary oedema. The best combination of drugs in acute myocardial infarction is aspirin and streptokinase. Aspirin prevents any new clots forming with its antiplatelet action and streptokinase breaks any existing clots. β-blockers reduce the chronotropic and inotropic effect of the heart and this is not desirable.

7.13 Diabetes

1. H Low-dose aspirin
2. I Metformin
3. C Glibenclamide
4. K Short-acting insulin
5. G Low-calorie diabetic diet with low-sodium diet and exercise

If a patient is not responding to treatment with oral hypoglycaemics, long-acting insulin can be used. Metformin is the initial drug of choice, and it is often combined with glibenclamide or the newer drug rosiglitazone. Glibenclamide is the drug of choice in patients with renal failure. The first step after giving a diagnosis of type 2 diabetes is to advise the patient regarding diet and exercise, as this can often be an effective treatment for this condition.

7.14 Antibiotics (1)

1. I Oral nitrofurantoin
2. E Flucloxacillin and fusidic acid
3. F Intravenous cefuroxime
4. D Erythromycin and amoxicillin
5. B Cefotaxime

Women are more susceptible than men to urinary tract infections, and some may need to take prophylactic antibiotics. The initial treatment for community-acquired pneumonia in the UK is surprisingly simple. Amoxicillin and erythromycin are a good combination of drugs until cultures are grown. Cefotaxime is the drug of choice if meningitis is suspected.

7.15 Adverse Drug Reactions

1 H Simvastatin

2 B Digoxin

3 I Verapamil

4 C Doxazosin

5 J Warfarin

Simvastatin is taken to lower cholesterol and has two main side-effects – derangement of liver function and myositis. Doxazosin is an α-channel blocker and common side-effects are dizziness, light-headedness and a drop in postural blood pressure. Patients who have atrial fibrillation are commonly prescribed digoxin and warfarin, and you need to know their side-effects. Patients may over-medicate with warfarin, and this can lead to bleeding.

7.16 Acute Asthma and Chronic Obstructive Pulmonary Disease (COPD)

1 F Nebulised salbutamol and ipratropium bromide, 60% oxygen, intravenous hydrocortisone and intravenous aminophylline

2 C Intravenous chlorphenamine, intramuscular adrenaline and intravenous hydrocortisone

3 J Nebulised salbutamol, 40% oxygen and prednisolone

4 L Salbutamol infusion

5 B Broad-spectrum antibiotics, nebulised salbutamol, ipratropium bromide, oral prednisolone and 28% oxygen

The above scenarios relate to the correct management for acute severe asthma, life-threatening asthma and anaphylaxis. Aminophylline should be avoided in pregnancy.

7.17 Practical Prescribing

1 J Surgical appliance request form

2 F Inpatient prescription chart – once-only medication

3 D Inpatient prescription chart – drugs with variable dosing schedules

4 G Inpatient prescription chart – regular medication

5 E Inpatient prescription chart – intravenous drugs with drug additives

Knowing where to prescribe on an inpatient drug chart is an important skill to learn.

7.18 Asthma and COPD

1 B Inhaled beclometasone

2 K Oral theophylline

3 C Inhaled ipratropium bromide

4 L Salbutamol via metered-dose inhaler

5 D Inhaled salmeterol

Patients who have asthma should be initially treated with salbutamol via a metered-dose inhaler. If their symptoms are not alleviated, they should use a beclometasone inhaler, and possibly salmeterol (long-acting β_2-agonist). After this oral steroids and theophyllines should be considered. Patients with COPD require bronchodilatation. β_2-agonists and antimuscarinics such as ipratropium bromide should be used for this. Oral theophyllines may be used for acute phase, but they have side-effects.

7.19 Overdose

1 B Activated charcoal only

2 F Flumazenil intravenously

3 E Atropine intravenously

4 J Naloxone

5 K N-acetylcysteine intravenously

7.20 Drug Interaction

1 D Diarrhoea

2 E Dyspnoea and wheeze

3 C Postural hypotension

4 H Neutropenia

5 B Constipation

Misoprostol and diclofenac lead to diarrhoea. Use of a β-blocker (timolol) in asthmatic patients leads to bronchoconstriction and therefore dyspnoea and wheeze. Patients on chemotherapy tend to have bone marrow suppression and therefore neutropenia. Dihydrocodeine belongs to the opiate family and leads to constipation.

7.21 Drugs and the Liver

1 F Methotrexate

2 A Alcohol

3 H Simvastatin

4 C Codeine phosphate

5 G Rifampicin

Methotrexate is a valuable drug in patients with rheumatoid arthritis, but they should be monitored for lung fibrosis. Simvastatin causes derangement of liver function. Codeine leads to constipation, and it is metabolised in the liver. However, in a patient with liver failure, it will not be metabolised and the opiate side-effect of central nervous system depression will occur. Rifampicin prevents the function of the oral contraceptive pill.

7.22 Drugs and Misuse

1 C Crack cocaine

2 G LSD

3 B Cannabis

4 F Ketamine

5 E Heroin

There are many different drugs which are abused by patients. They are used more commonly than most dental students think. It is important to have knowledge of these drugs and their interactions with prescribed drugs.

PHARMACOLOGY

7.23 Polypharmacy

1 J Verapamil

2 E Metolazone

3 I Spironolactone

4 G Prednisolone

5 D Erythromycin

Verapamil is a calcium channel blocker and can lead to heart block; spironolactone is a potassium-sparing diuretic, and will therefore lead to a build up of potassium, and metolazone does the opposite. Erythromycin interacts with warfarin and can lead to a rise in the INR.

7.24 Drugs and Pregnancy (2)

1 E Chlorphenamine

2 J Low-molecular-weight heparin

3 D Cefuroxime

4 C Carbimazole

5 K Methyldopa

Warfarin is teratogenic, therefore heparin is preferable in pregnancy. Cefuroxime is safe in pregnancy. Radioactive iodine is contraindicated, but carbimazole is safe. Angiotensin-converting enzyme (ACE) inhibitors should not be used to treat hypertension in pregnancy, but methyldopa is safe.

7.25 Statistical Terminology

1	F	Positive predictive value
2	I	Specificity
3	A	Confidence interval
4	E	Number needed to treat
5	H	Sensitivity

There is a greater emphasis on statistics in dentistry today. A knowledge of this is required to be able to interpret data from scientific papers.

7.26 Clinical Trials

1	K	Subgroup analysis
2	D	Double blind
3	G	Real end point
4	A	Absolute risk reduction
5	L	Surrogate end point

Knowledge of statistical terminology is required to be able to evaluate the efficacy of treatment and understand scientific papers.

7.27 Treatment of Arthritis

| 1 | F | Ibuprofen and ranitidine |

| 2 | C | Celecoxib |

| 3 | I | Methotrexate and folic acid |

| 4 | D | Colchicine |

| 5 | K | Prednisolone |

Rheumatoid arthritis is a progressive arthropathy which requires complex treatment. Methotrexate is effective but has side-effects of pulmonary and liver fibrosis, so must be used sparingly. In gout, acute phases are managed with colchicine and prophylaxis is with allopurinol. Treatment of acute polymyalgia rheumatica is with steroids.

7.28 Common Arrhythmias

| 1 | G | Verapamil |

| 2 | F | Oral amiodarone |

| 3 | I | Warfarin for life |

| 4 | D | DC cardioversion |

| 5 | H | Warfarin for 4 weeks |

To restore a rhythm such as ventricular tachycardia, DC cardioversion is required, but prophylaxis can be provided by oral amiodarone. Patients with permanent atrial fibrillation require warfarin prophylaxis to prevent thrombus/embolus formation.

7.29 Antibiotics (2)

1 A Amoxicillin

2 C Clindamycin

3 H Metronidazole

4 F Gentamicin

5 A Amoxicillin

8 Radiology

8.1 Theme: Frequency of Taking Radiographs to Monitor Dental Disease
8.2 Theme: Selection of Radiographic Views
8.3 Theme: Component Parts of an Intra-Oral X-Ray Set
8.4 Theme: Multilocular Radiolucencies at the Angle of the Mandible
8.5 Theme: Odontogenic Cysts (1)
8.6 Theme: Odontogenic Cysts (2)
8.7 Theme: Odontogenic Cysts (3)
8.8 Theme: Odontogenic Cysts (4)
8.9 Theme: Oral Tumours (1)
8.10 Theme: Oral Tumours (2)
8.11 Theme: Oral Tumours (3)
8.12 Theme: Oral Tumours (4)
8.13 Theme: Facial Fractures (1)
8.14 Theme: Facial Fractures (2)
8.15 Theme: Bone Lesions
8.16 Theme: Benign Tumours
8.17 Theme: Radiological Diagnosis
8.18 Theme: Non-Odontogenic Cysts
8.19 Theme: Malignant Tumours (1)
8.20 Theme: Malignant Tumours (2)
8.21 Theme: Oral Tumours (5)
8.22 Theme: More Cysts
8.23 Theme: Salivary Glands
8.24 Theme: Trauma (1)
8.25 Theme: Trauma (2)
8.26 Theme: Oral Tumours (6)

8.1 Theme: Frequency of Taking Radiographs to Monitor Dental Disease

A 3-monthly
B 6-monthly
C 12-monthly
D 18-monthly
E 24-monthly
F 30-monthly

For each of the following clinical scenarios, choose the recommended frequency of radiographic review from the list above. You may use each option once, more than once or not at all.

1. A 3-year-old with multiple carious lesions evident.
2. An adult with multiple carious lesions evident.
3. An adult who has recently had a molar tooth root filled.
4. Non-restored dentition with no caries evident in an adult.

8.2 Theme: Selection of Radiographic Views

A Bitewing
B Dental panoramic tomogram
C Occlusal
D Periapical
E Lateral skull
F Occipitomental

For each of the assessments below, choose the most appropriate image from the list above. You may use each option once, more than once or not at all.

1. Orthodontic skull analysis.
2. Working length radiograph for an incisor.
3. Diagnosing approximal caries in premolars.
4. Third molar assessment.
5. Molar with 6 mm deep pocket.

8.3 Theme: Component Parts of an Intra-Oral X-ray Set

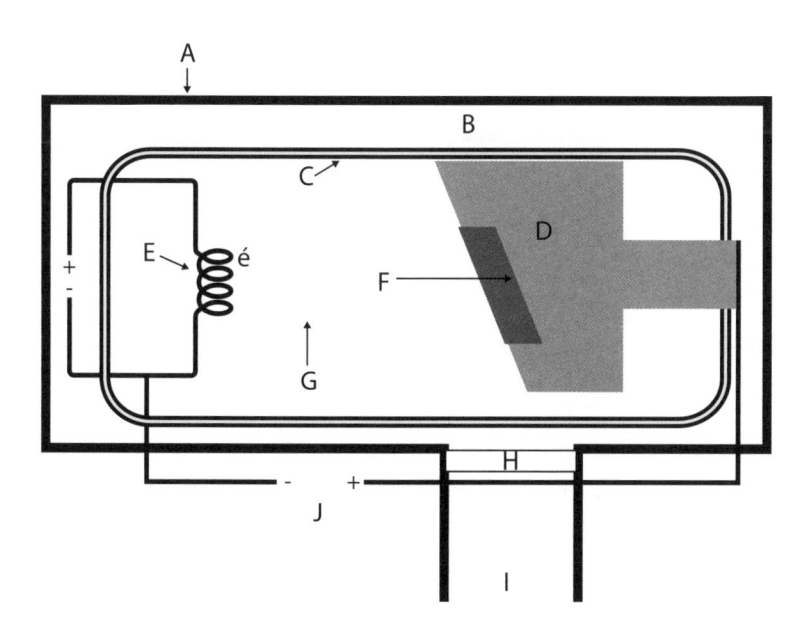

Look at the diagram above of an intra-oral X-ray set. For each of the following descriptions, choose the most appropriate labelled option from the diagram. You may use each option once, more than once or not at all.

1 Aluminium filter
2 Filament
3 Inert gas filled space
4 Oil filled space
5 Tungsten target

8.4 Theme: Multilocular Radiolucencies at the Angle of the Mandible

A   Ameloblastoma
B   Aneurysmal bone cyst
C   Brown's tumour
D   Cherubism
E   Odontogenic keratocyst

For each of the following scenarios, select the most appropriate option from the list above. You may use each option once, more than once or not at all.

1   A 12-year-old child presents with facial fullness, and an orthopantomogram (OPG) shows bilateral mandibular multilocular radiolucencies at the angle of the mandible.

2   A patient on the renal ward is referred to you with an abnormal dental X-ray by the renal team. He has hypercalcaemia, which is currently under investigation. The renal team has queried a bone malignancy of the mandible.

3   A 21-year-old woman is referred by her dentist for surgical extraction of her wisdom teeth by your surgical department. On examination you detect a swelling with a bluish discoloration of the gingiva of the lower right quadrant. An OPG shows horizontally impacted lower wisdom teeth with a multilocular radiolucency on the right. She says the swelling increases at the time of her period.

4   An African man presents with minimal external swelling but a large radiographic lesion. He complains of loose teeth and on palpation of the buccal cortex there is 'egg shell crackling'.

5   At the time of removal of a patient's lower right third molar you sent some abnormal follicular material to the histopathology laboratory. The report says the cyst has a daughter cyst in the cystic membrane.

RADIOLOGY   303

8.5   Theme: Odontogenic Cysts (1)

A	Dentigerous cyst	K	Round
B	Radicular cyst	L	Oval
C	Odontogenic keratocyst	M	Square
D	Rests of Malassez	N	No normal shape
E	Glands of Serres	O	Mesio-distal
F	Enamel organ	P	Medio-lateral
G	1%	Q	Does not expand
H	5%		
I	25%		
J	50%		

For each of the following questions regarding the figure below, choose the most appropriate option from the list above. You may use each option once, more than once or not at all.

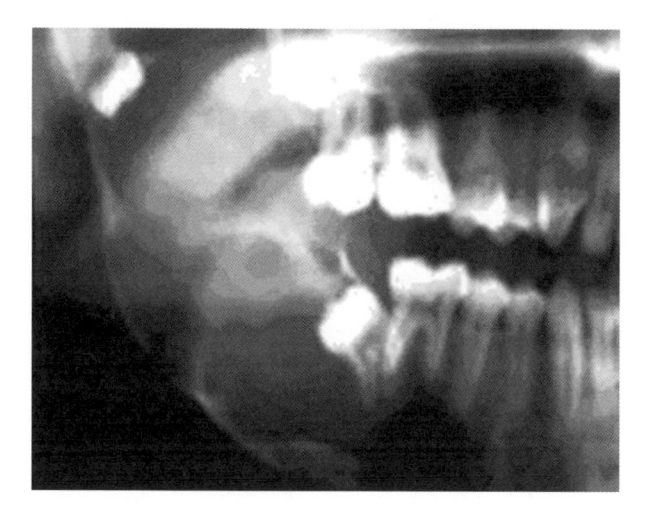

1. What is the diagnosis?
2. What epithelial remnant does it develop from?
3. What proportion of odontogenic cysts do they form?
4. What is the classic shape?
5. In which direction does it expand?

8.6 Theme: Odontogenic Cysts (2)

A	Radiodense
B	Radiolucent
C	Both radiodense and radiolucent
D	1–10 years
E	20–40 years
F	40–60 years
G	60+ years
H	Anterior mandible
I	Anterior maxilla
J	Posterior maxilla
K	Addison's disease
L	Gorlin–Goltz syndrome
M	Kallmann syndrome
N	Basal cell carcinoma
O	Squamous cell carcinoma
P	Ameloblastoma

For each of the following questions regarding the figure in question 8.5, choose the most appropriate option from the list above. You may use each option once, more than once or not at all.

1. How would you describe the appearance of the lesion?
2. In which age range is it usually discovered?
3. Other than the posterior mandible, what area of the mouth is it found in most commonly?
4. Which syndrome is this lesion associated with?
5. What cancer is the syndrome in Q 4 associated with?

8.7 Theme: Odontogenic Cysts (3)

A	Idiopathic bone cyst
B	Radicular cyst
C	Dentigerous cyst
D	Lateral periodontal cyst
E	0-18 years
F	18-40 years
G	40-60 years
H	60+ years
I	Mandibular third permanent molars
J	Mandibular premolars
K	Maxillary third permanent molars
L	Maxillary canines
M	Gingival cyst
N	Eruption cyst

For each of the following questions regarding the figure below, choose the most appropriate option from the list above. You may use each option once, more than once or not at all.

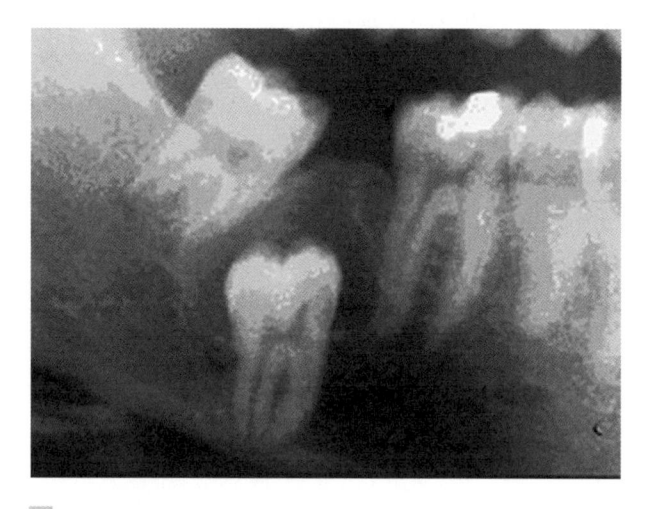

1. What is the diagnosis?
2. In which age range is this condition usually diagnosed?
3. Which teeth are most commonly affected by this condition?
4. Which teeth are the next most commonly affected?
5. If this cyst caused a clinically visible swelling in the gingival region, what would it be called?

8.8 Theme: Odontogenic Cysts (4)

A   Root
B   Enamel
C   Amelocemental junction
D   Dentine
E   Radiolucent
F   Radiopaque
G   Mixed
H   Intra-oral peri-apical (IOPA)
I   Postero-anterior (PA) mandible
J   Orthopantomogram (OPG)
K   Displaced
L   Resorbed
M   Both
N   1%
O   5%
P   25%
Q   60%

For each of the following questions regarding the figure in Q 8.7, choose the most appropriate option from the list above. You may use each option once, more than once or not at all.

1. Where on the tooth is this cyst usually attached?
2. How would you describe the appearance of the lesion?
3. What is the best X-ray to diagnose this condition?
4. What usually happens to adjacent teeth?
5. What proportion of all odontogenic cysts does this form?

8.9 Theme: Oral Tumours (1)

A	Calcified epithelial odontogenic tumour
B	Cemento-ossifying fibroma
C	True cementoma
D	0–18 years
E	18–40 years
F	40–60 years
G	60+ years
H	0–1 cm
I	1–3 cm
J	3–7 cm
K	7+ cm
L	Mandibular molars
M	Maxillary molars
N	Mandibular anterior teeth
O	Maxillary anterior teeth
P	Well defined
Q	Poorly defined
R	No pattern

For each of the following questions regarding the figure below, choose the most appropriate option from the list above. You may use each option once, more than once or not at all.

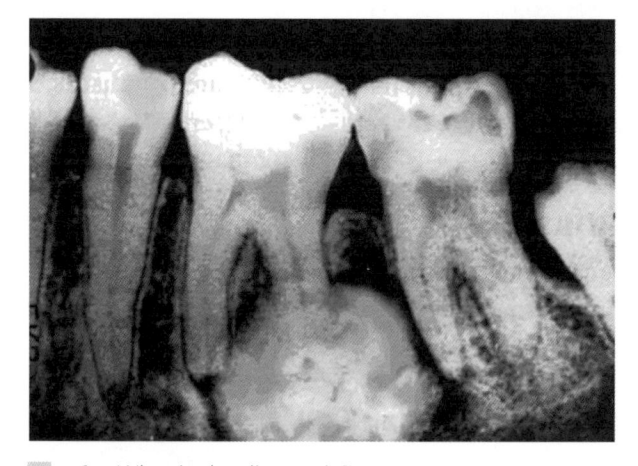

1. What is the diagnosis?
2. When is it usually discovered?
3. What is the usual size of this lesion?
4. To which teeth is it most commonly attached?
5. What is the pattern to the definition of the lesion?

8.10 Theme: Oral Tumours (2)

A	Radiolucent
B	Radiopaque
C	Mixed radiolucent/radiopaque
D	Benign
E	Locally invasive
F	Malignant
G	Golf ball
H	Rugby ball
I	Tennis ball
J	Mandibular molars
K	Maxillary molars
L	Maxillary anteriors
M	Mandibular anteriors
N	Male
O	Female
P	Affects males as frequently as females

For each of the following questions regarding the figure in Q 8.9, choose the most appropriate option from the list above. You may use each option once, more than once or not at all.

1. What is the appearance of the lesion?
2. What is the behaviour of the lesion?
3. What is the classical description of the shape of the lesion?
4. If this lesion was periapical cemento-osseous dysplasia rather than a true cementum, which teeth would it affect?
5. Which sex is affected more commonly?

8.11 Theme: Oral Tumours (3)

A	Calcifying epithelial odontogenic tumour	I	Posterior mandible
		J	Posterior maxilla
B	Central giant cell granuloma	K	Anterior mandible
C	Fibrous dysplasia	L	Anterior maxilla
D	Radicular cyst	M	Monolocular
E	0–18 years	N	Multilocular
F	18–30 years	O	No pattern
G	30–50 years	P	Smooth and undulating
H	50+ years	Q	Irregular and always well defined

For each of the following questions regarding the figure below, choose the most appropriate option from the list above. You may use each option once, more than once or not at all.

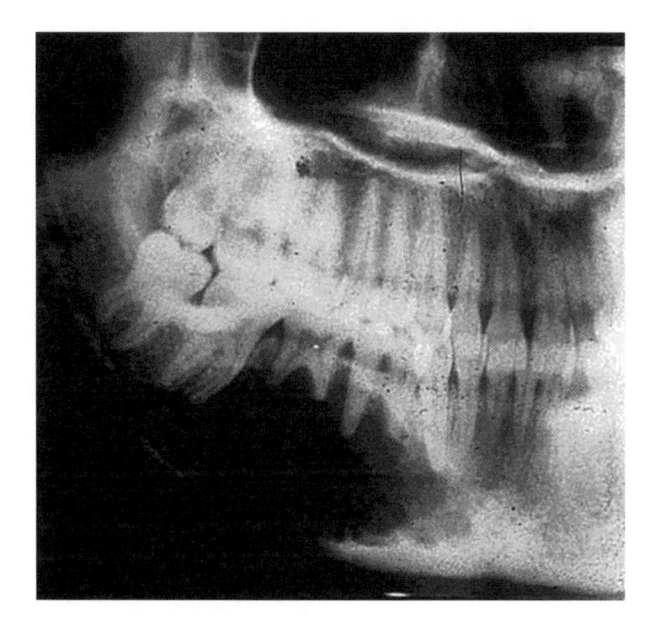

1. What is the diagnosis?
2. In which age group is this most commonly detected?
3. In which region of the jaws is this most commonly detected?
4. How would you describe the appearance of the lesion?
5. What is the outline like?

8.12 Theme: Oral Tumours (4)

A Radiopaque
B Radiolucent
C Mixed lucency
D Sunray
E Honeycomb
F Mosaic
G Mesio-distal expansion
H Bucco-lingual expansion
I Does not expand
J Hyperthyroidism
K Hypothyroidism
L Hyperparathyroidism
M Hypoparathyroidism
N Cherubism
O Familial gigantiform cementoma
P Gardner syndrome

For each of the following questions regarding the figure in Q 8.11, choose the most appropriate option from the list above. You may use each option once, more than once or not at all.

1. How would you describe the appearance of this lesion?
2. What is the textbook description of the lesion?
3. Describe the direction of expansion of this lesion.
4. Giant cell lesions are associated with which endocrinopathy?
5. What is the name of the rare giant cell lesion which is autosomal dominant, appears in children between 2 and 6 years old and causes extensive disfigurement because of its rapidly expanding multilocular lesions?

8.13 Theme: Facial Fractures (1)

A Fractured mandible
B Fractured zygoma
C Le Fort I fracture
D Le Fort II fracture
E Occipito-mental (OM) 0° and OM 30°
F OM 10° and OM 50°
G OM 30° and OM 70°
H Left
I Right
J Occurs equally on the left and right
K Car accidents
L Interpersonal trauma
M Sport
N Work-related injury
O Winter
P Campbell
Q Jones

For each of the following questions regarding the figures below, choose the most appropriate option from the list above. You may use each option once, more than once or not at all.

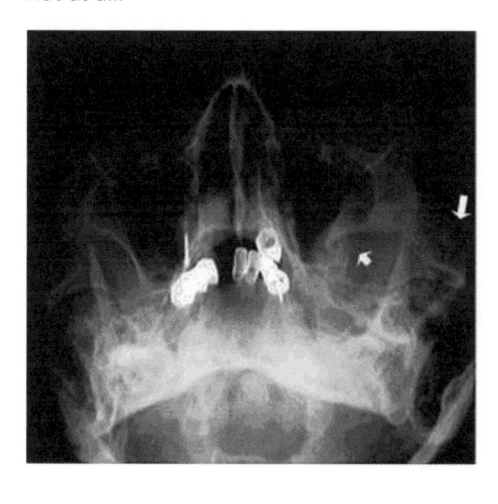

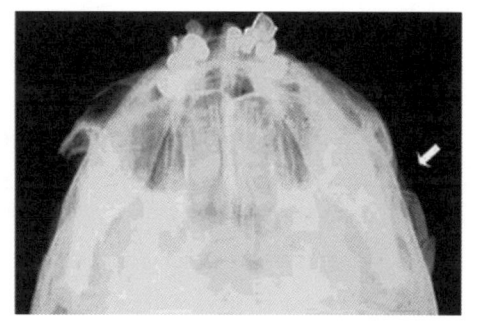

1. What is the diagnosis?
2. Which X-rays are these?
3. On which side of the face does this lesion usually occur?
4. What is the most common cause of this lesion?
5. What lines should you follow when interpreting the above X-ray?

8.14 Theme: Facial Fractures (2)

A Masseter
B Temporalis
C Lateral pterygoid
D Medial pterygoid
E Hooper's forceps
F Gillies' hook
G McIndoe
H Howarth's elevator
I Facial
J Inferior-dental
K Infra-orbital
L Supra-trochlear
M Clear
N Narrowed
O Cloudy
P Have you ever had this condition before?
Q Have you lost consciousness?
R Can you feel your cheek?

For each of the following questions regarding the figures in Q 8.13, choose the most appropriate option from the list above. You may use each option once, more than once or not at all.

1. Which muscle inserts into the anterior two-thirds of the bone indicated by the arrows?
2. Which eponymous instrument is used to correct this problem?
3. Which nerve is frequently affected by paraesthesia or anaesthesia in this condition?
4. What is the common appearance of the antrum in this condition?
5. What question should be asked initially if a patient presents acutely with this condition?

8.15 Theme: Bone Lesions

A	Multiple myeloma	H	Sunray
B	Osteomyelitis	I	Moth-eaten
C	Paget's disease	J	Burnt leaf
D	Involucrum	K	Maxilla
E	Sequestrum	L	Mandible
F	Partition	M	Temporal bone
G	Cortical reformation	N	Occipital bone

For each of the following questions regarding the figures below, choose the most appropriate option from the list above. You may use each option once, more than once or not at all.

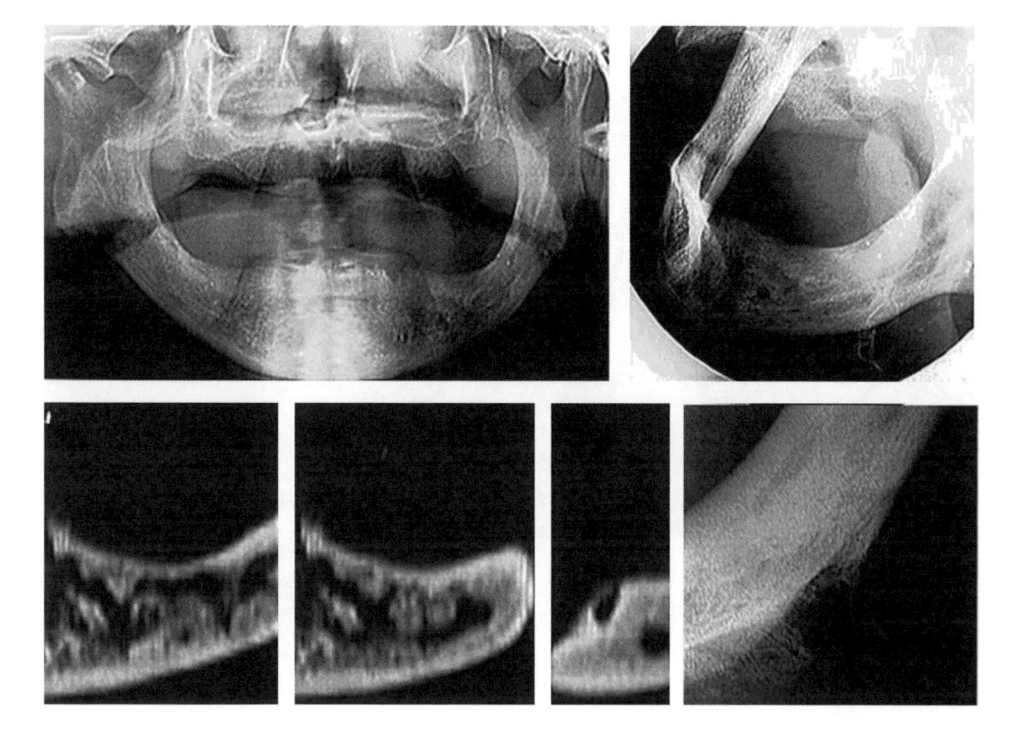

1 What is the diagnosis?
2 Which is the name of the dead bone in this condition?
3 What is the name of the newly formed bone in this condition?
4 What is the textbook description of the radiographic lesion?
5 Where does it most commonly occur in the skull?

8.16 Theme: Benign Tumours

A	Ameloblastoma	J	Maxilla
B	Benign cementoma	K	Occipital bone
C	Fibrous dysplasia	L	Frontal bone
D	Squamous cell carcinoma	M	Anterior
E	0-10 years	N	Mid-section
F	10-20 years	O	Posterior
G	20-30 years	P	Round
H	30-40 years	Q	Square
I	Mandible	R	Triangular

For each of the following questions regarding the figures below, choose the most appropriate option from the list above. You may use each option once, more than once or not at all.

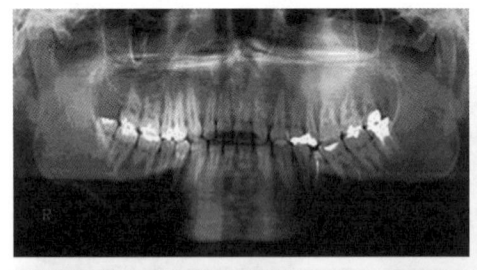

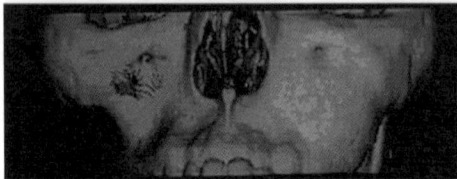

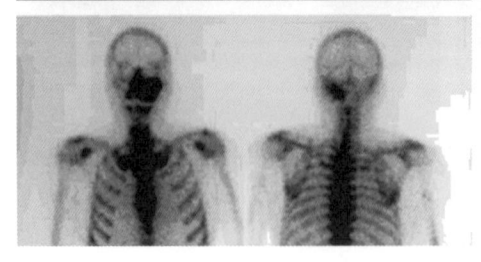

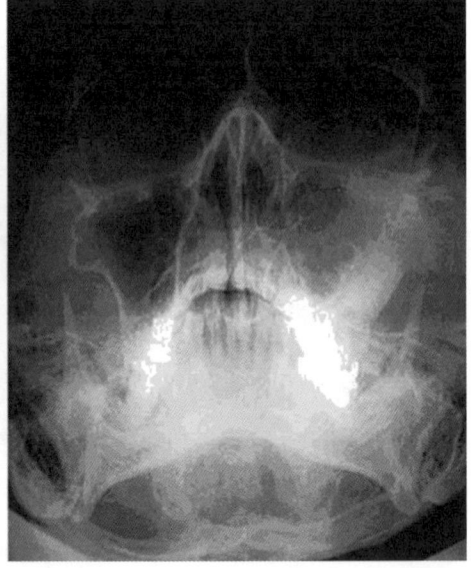

1 What is the diagnosis?
2 In which age group is this condition most prevalent?
3 In which bone of the skull is this most prevalent?
4 In which region of the bone does it most commonly occur?
5 What is the typical shape of the lesion?

8.17 Theme: Radiological Diagnosis

A   Poorly defined
B   Well defined
C   Could be well defined or poorly defined
D   Computed tomography (CT)
E   Magnetic resonance imaging (MRI)
F   Positron emission tomography (PET)
G   Radiopaque
H   Radiolucent
I   Mixed radiopaque and radiolucent
J   Ivory
K   Orange peel
L   Sunray
M   Bucco-lingual
N   Mesio-distal
O   Does not expand

For each of the following questions regarding the figures in Q 8.16, choose the most appropriate option from the list above. You may use each option once, more than once or not at all.

1   Describe the definition of this lesion.
2   What type of scan is shown in the lowermost picture?
3   How would you describe the lucency/opacity of this lesion?
4   What is the classic radiographic description of this condition?
5   In which direction does the lesion expand?

RADIOLOGY

8.18 Theme: Non-Odontogenic Cysts

A	Adenocystic carcinoma	K	10%
B	Aneurysmal bone cyst	L	20%
C	Nasopalatine duct cyst	M	Anterior maxilla
D	Radicular cyst	N	Mid-maxilla
E	0–20 years	O	Posterior maxilla
F	20–40 years	P	Smooth and well defined
G	40–60 years	Q	Smooth and poorly defined
H	60+ years	R	Rough and well defined
I	0.1%	S	Rough and poorly defined
J	1%		

For each of the following questions regarding the figures below, choose the most appropriate option from the list above. Please note that in this case, all of the maxillary anterior teeth are vital. You may use each option once, more than once or not at all.

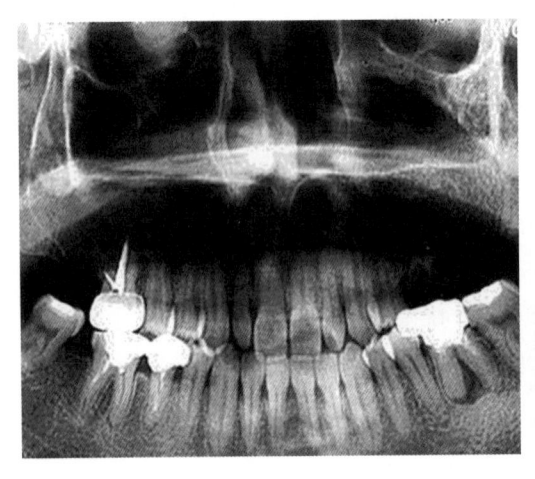

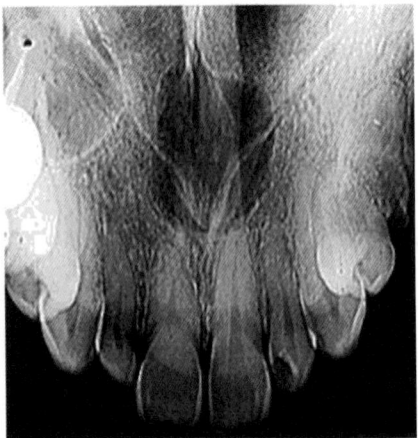

1. What is the diagnosis?
2. In which age group is this condition most commonly detected?
3. What percentage of the total population does this occur in?
4. Where does this condition usually occur?
5. What is the outline of the lesion usually like?

8.19 Theme: Malignant Tumours (1)

A	Hyperparathyroidism	I	Maxilla
B	Multiple myeloma	J	Hands
C	Paget's disease	K	0–20 years
D	Thalassaemia	L	20–40 years
E	Male	M	40–60 years
F	Female	N	60+ years
G	Equally prevalent in males and females	O	African-Caribbean
		P	Asian
H	Skull vault	Q	Caucasian

For each of the following questions regarding the figure below, choose the most appropriate option from the list above. You may use each option once, more than once or not at all.

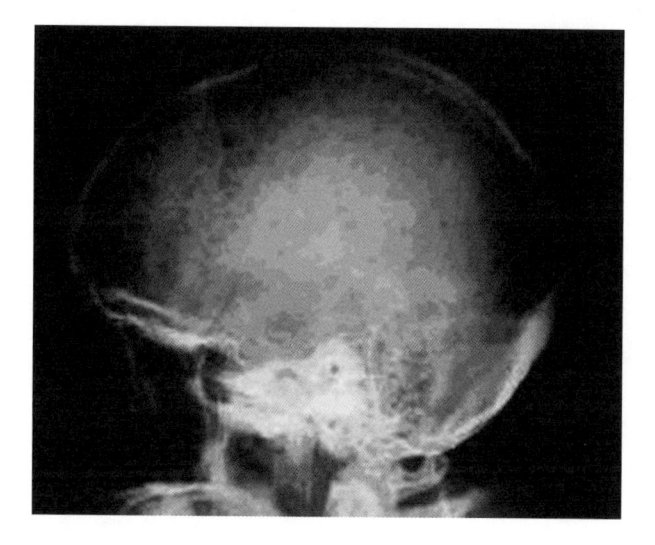

1 What is the diagnosis?
2 In which sex is this condition most prevalent?
3 Where is this condition most commonly found?
4 In which age group is this condition usually found?
5 In which ethnic group is this condition most prevalent?

8.20 Theme: Malignant Tumours (2)

A	Plasma cells
B	Red blood cells
C	Osteoblasts
D	Osteoclasts
E	Hair-on-end appearance
F	Pepper pot skull
G	Sunray appearance
H	Radiolucent
I	Radiopaque
J	Mixed lucency
K	Monolocular
L	Multilocular
M	Could be either monolocular or multilocular
N	Bence Jones
O	Clarke
P	Williams

For each of the following questions regarding the figure in Q 8.19, choose the most appropriate option from the list above. You may use each option once, more than once or not at all.

1. Which cells cause this condition?
2. What is the classic radiographic appearance of this condition?
3. Describe the lucency/opacity of this lesion.
4. Describe the locularity of the lesion.
5. Which protein is detected in the urine in this condition?

8.21 Theme: Oral Tumours (5)

A Odontogenic fibroma
B Normal anatomy
C Compound odontome
D Complex odontome
E Ameloblastoma
F Ossifying fibroma

For each of the following questions regarding the figures below, choose the most appropriate option from the list above. You may use each option once, more than once or not at all.

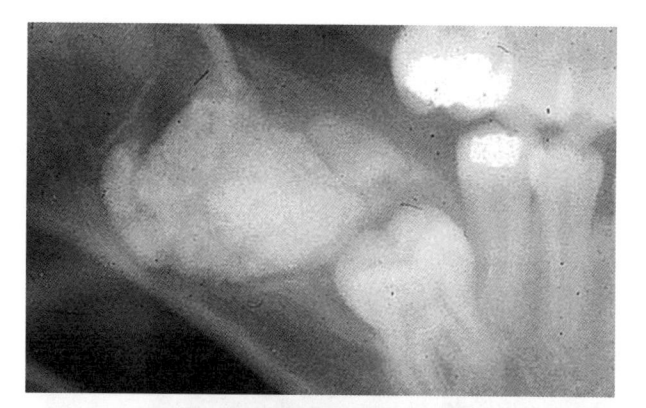

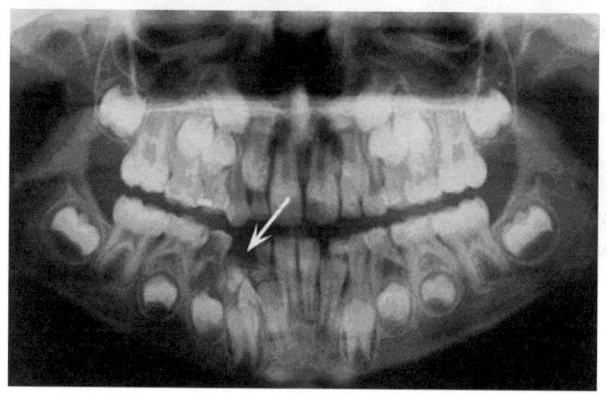

1 What is the diagnosis for the top image?
2 What is the diagnosis for the bottom image?

8.22 Theme: More Cysts

A	Ameloblastoma	N	Buccal
B	Eruption cyst	O	Palatal/lingual
C	Radicular cyst	P	Mesial/distal
D	Male	Q	5%
E	Female	R	25%
F	Equally prevalent in both sexes	S	75%
G	It is a developmental lesion	T	Rests of Malassez
H	Acquired via trauma	U	Glands of Serres
I	Malignant change	V	Enamel organ
J	Anterior mandible	W	Monolocular
K	Posterior mandible	X	Multilocular
L	Anterior maxilla	Y	Could be both monolocular or multilocular
M	Posterior maxilla		

For each of the following questions regarding the figures below, choose the most appropriate option from the list above. You may use each option once, more than once or not at all.

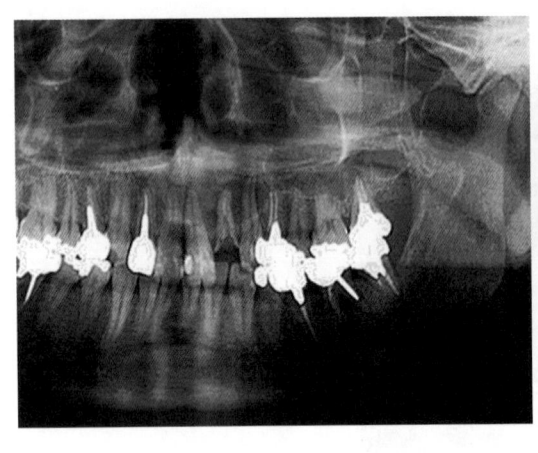

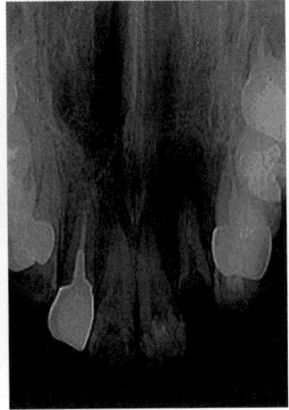

1. What is the diagnosis?
2. In which sex is this condition most prevalent?
3. What is the most common aetiological cause of this condition?
4. Where in the mouth is this condition most prevalent?
5. In which direction does this lesion expand?
6. What proportion of all jaw cysts does this lesion form?
7. What embryological remnant does this lesion form from?
8. Describe the locularity of the lesion.

8.23 Theme: Salivary Glands

A	Salivary calculi	I	Parotid gland
B	Adenoid cystic carcinoma	J	Submandibular gland
C	Pleomorphic adenoma	K	Sublingual gland
D	Sjögren syndrome	L	Sunray
E	Sialography	M	Snow storm
F	Plain film	N	Tree in winter
G	CT scanning	O	Osteoarthritis
H	PET scanning	P	Rheumatoid arthritis
		Q	Sero-negative arthritis

For each of the following questions regarding the figures below, choose the most appropriate option from the list above. You may use each option once, more than once or not at all.

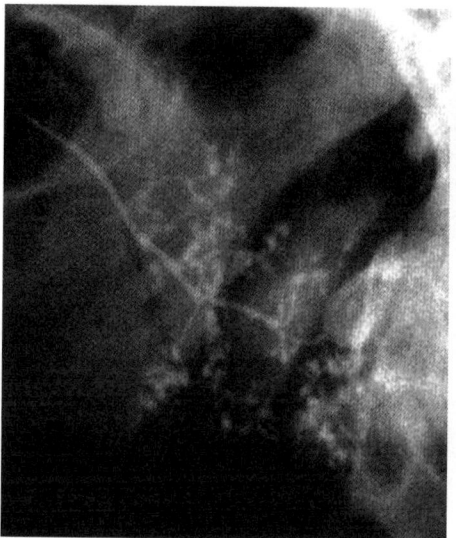

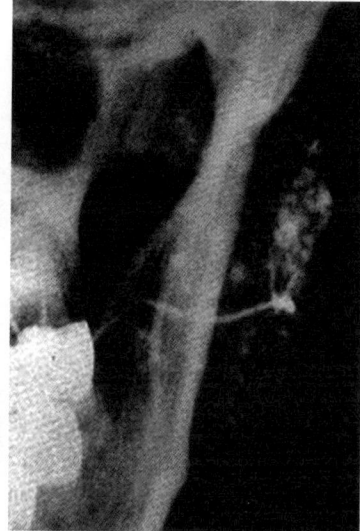

1. What is the diagnosis?
2. What type of radiography is this?
3. Which anatomical site is this X-ray showing?
4. What is the classic textbook description of this condition?
5. What other degenerative condition is this condition associated with?

8.24 Theme: Trauma (1)

A	Fractured mandible	J	MRI
B	Fractured zygomatic arch	K	Plain film
C	Fractured orbital floor	L	Cavernous sinus thrombosis
D	Fractured nasal bones	M	Airway difficulty
E	OPG	N	Retrobulbar haemorrhage
F	OM	O	Sunray
G	PA mandible	P	Hanging drop
H	AP mandible	Q	Pillar box
I	CT	R	Orange peel

For each of the following questions regarding the figures below, choose the most appropriate option from the list above. Please note that the images are not of the same person, but they show the same type of lesion. You may use each option once, more than once or not at all.

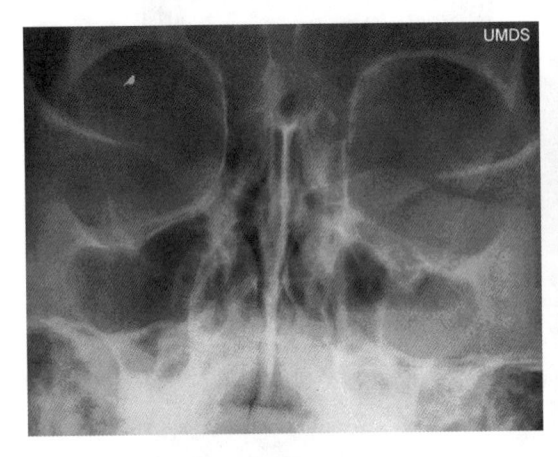

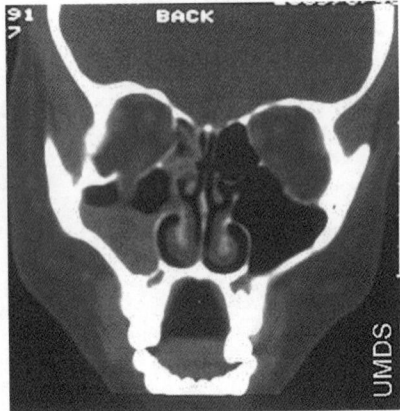

1. What is the diagnosis?
2. What radiographic view is seen in the left figure?
3. What type of radiography is seen in the right figure?
4. What medical emergency is this injury associated with?
5. What classic radiographic sign is seen in both films?

8.25 Theme: Trauma (2)

A   Subconjunctival haematoma
B   Enophthalmos
C   Exophthalmos
D   Trismus
E   Diplopia
F   Inability to feel maxillary teeth
G   Proptosis
H   Interpersonal trauma
I   Work-related injury
J   Road traffic accident
K   Retinal detachment
L   Temporal arteritis
M   Damage to the infra-orbital nerve
N   Blow your nose to clear your sinuses
O   Do not blow your nose
P   Wear an eye patch
Q   Eat a soft diet

For each of the following questions regarding the figures in Q 8.24, choose the most appropriate option from the list above. You may use each option once, more than once or not at all.

1. What is the term given to the sunken-in appearance of the eye after this injury?
2. What is the most common patient complaint with this lesion?
3. What is the most common cause of this injury?
4. If a patient complains of 'floaters' and difficulty with bright light, what diagnosis should you be considering?
5. If you suspect this lesion, what cautionary advice would you give to the patient?

8.26 Theme: Oral Tumours (6)

A   Ameloblastoma
B   Fractured mandible
C   Stafne's idiopathic bone cyst
D   0–18 years
E   18–35 years
F   35–50 years
G   50+ years
H   Posterior mandible
I   Anterior mandible
J   Posterior maxilla
K   Anterior maxilla
L   Monolocular
M   Multilocular
N   Can be either monolocular or multilocular
O   Orange peel
P   Soap bubble
Q   Sunray

For each of the following questions regarding the figure below, choose the most appropriate option from the list above. You may use each option once, more than once or not at all.

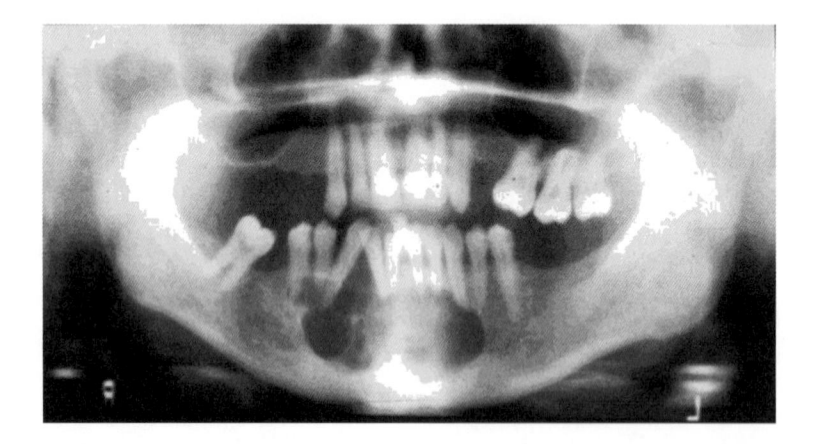

1. What is the diagnosis?
2. In which age group does this lesion usually occur?
3. Where does it usually occur?
4. Describe the locularity of the lesion.
5. What is the classic radiographic description of this lesion?

8.1 Frequency of Taking Radiographs to Monitor Dental Disease

1 B 6-monthly

2 B 6-monthly

3 C 12-monthly

4 E 24-monthly

High caries risk children show have posterior bitewing radiographs every six months until no new or active lesions are apparent and the individual has entered another risk category. Bitewings should not be taken more frequently and it is imperative to reassess caries risk in order to justify using this interval again.

Low caries risk children should be radiographed at approximately 12–18-month intervals in the primary dentition and approximately 24-month intervals for the secondary dentition.

The European Academy of Paediatric Dentistry (EAPD) have different guidelines to the Faculty of General Dental Practice (UK) and recommend only 36-monthly posterior bitewing examination in low caries risk children.

It is recommended that for an adult who recently has had a molar tooth root treated a 12-monthly radiographic follow-up should be conducted and compared to the filled radiograph taken at the time of root filling. At one year, radiographic evidence of healing of an apical area should be present.

Adults with a low caries risk are recommended to have posterior bitewings no frequently than 24-monthly.

Reference: "Selection Criteria for dental Radiography" by the Faculty of General Dental Practice (UK) 3rd Edition 2013

ANSWERS

8.2 Selection of Radiographic Views

| 1 | E | Lateral skull |

| 2 | D | Periapical |

| 3 | A | Bitewing |

| 4 | B | Dental panoramic tomogram |

| 5 | D | Periapical |

Cephalometric analysis is done with a lateral skull view.

Bitewings are good for diagnosing approximal caries and early bone loss in periodontitis. Endodontics requires a periapical view as well as more advanced periodontal diseases.

Third molars, especially if extraction is being considered, are best assessed by dental panoramic tomogram as local anatomy can also be assessed, crucially the apex and location of the inferior alveolar nerve canal.

8.3 Component Parts of an Intra-Oral X-ray Set

| 1 | H | Aluminium filter |

| 2 | E | Filament |

| 3 | G | Inert gas filled space |

| 4 | B | Oil filled space |

| 5 | F | Tungsten target |

Other parts labelled are:

A   Metal box
C   Glass envelope
D   Copper block
I   Collimator
J   Kilovolt peak kVp

RADIOLOGY

8.4 Multilocular Radiolucencies at the Angle of the Mandible

1 D Cherubism

2 C Brown's tumour

3 B Aneurysmal bone cyst

4 A Ameloblastoma

5 E Odontogenic keratocyst

The differential diagnosis for a multilocular radiolucency within the jaws can include numerous conditions. The odontogenic keratocyst and ameloblastoma are the most common considerations, and both of these lesions exhibit a predilection for the posterior mandible. In addition, a central giant cell granuloma can appear in a similar manner, although this lesion tends to involve anterior portions of the jaws. Less common entities that can be included in the differential diagnosis are odontogenic myxoma, ameloblastic fibroma, central odontogenic fibroma and intraosseous mucoepidermoid carcinoma. A variety of additional rare entities, including odontogenic tumours, odontogenic cysts and other benign lesions, also can appear as a multilocular radiolucency. Because this radiographic pattern is not specific, a biopsy and histopathological examination are required to reach a definitive diagnosis.

8.5 Odontogenic Cysts (1)

1 C Odontogenic keratocyst

2 E Glands of Serres

3 H 5%

4 L Oval

5 P Medio-lateral

8.6 Odontogenic Cysts (2)

1 B Radiolucent

2 E 20–40 years

3 I Anterior maxilla

4 L Gorlin–Goltz syndrome

5 N Basal cell carcinoma

Odontogenic keratocysts are derived from the dental lamina, the cell glands of Serres, instead of the normal tooth, which is why there is often one tooth missing from the series. They are often discovered in the third decade, and comprise 5% of all odontogenic cysts. They are frequently found in the posterior mandible and in the maxillary canine region. They are often large in size and are classically oval in shape. They are either pseudo-locular or multilocular, with a smooth, well-defined, often well-corticated, outline. They are radiolucent, and cause minimal displacement of teeth. Resorption occurs rarely, but there is typically extensive expansion of the cancellous bone. Odontogenic keratocysts are associated with Gorlin–Goltz syndrome. This syndrome comprises cleidocranial dysplasia, calcified falx cerebri, multiple odontogenic keratocysts and basal cell naevi.

8.7 Odontogenic Cysts (3)

1 C Dentigerous cyst

2 E 0–18 years

3 I Mandibular third permanent molars

4 L Maxillary canines

5 N Eruption cyst

8.8 Odontogenic Cysts (4)

1	C	Amelocemental junction
2	E	Radiolucent
3	J	OPG
4	K	Displaced
5	P	25%

Dentigerous cysts develop from remnants of the reduced enamel epithelium after the tooth has formed. They are usually discovered when identifying the position of wisdom teeth. They account for a quarter of all odontogenic cysts. They are most commonly associated with unerupted teeth, and if they extend into the soft tissues above the unerupted tooth, they are called eruption cysts. They are round or oval cysts which envelope the crown and are attached to the amelodentinal junction. They are smooth, well defined and often well corticated. They are uniformly radiolucent, displace and rarely cause resorption of adjacent teeth.

8.9 Oral Tumours (1)

1	C	True cementoma
2	D	0–18 years
3	I	1–3 cm
4	L	Mandibular molars
5	P	Well defined

8.10 Oral Tumours (2)

1. B Radiopaque
2. D Benign
3. G Golf ball
4. M Mandibular anteriors
5. O Female

The true (benign) cementoma occurs always before the age of 25 years and most commonly in the under-18 age group. It occurs rarely, and is found at the apex of a root of a molar and sometimes a premolar. It is a round and irregular lesion, and attached to the root. It is classically described as having a 'golf ball' shape. It is a well-defined, radiopaque lesion, surrounded by a radiolucent halo. The lesion is actually fused to the tooth root, which is usually obscured as a result of resorption and fusion. If the lesion is large, it may cause cortical expansion. Periapical cemento-osseous dysplasia affects middle-aged women, and there are often multiple monolocular lesions attached to typically vital mandibular anterior teeth.

8.11 Oral Tumours (3)

1. B Central giant cell granuloma
2. F 18–30 years
3. K Anterior mandible
4. N Multilocular
5. P Smooth and undulating

8.12 Oral Tumours (4)

1	B	Radiolucent
2	E	Honeycomb
3	H	Bucco-lingual expansion
4	L	Hyperparathyroidism
5	N	Cherubism

The central giant cell granuloma is a non-neoplastic mass which produces an expansile radiolucent lesion in the jaws. It occurs in young adults under the age of 30 years. It most commonly occurs in the anterior mandible, often crossing the midline, and it can be up to 10 cm in diameter. It is a multilocular lesion with a smooth and undulating outline. Although it is radiolucent, larger lesions have interseptal trabeculae, which give it a honeycomb appearance. Anterior teeth are often displaced, and it expands bucco-lingually. Brown's tumours are associated with hyperparathyroidism, and cherubism is a rare giant cell condition affecting young children.

8.13 Facial Fractures (1)

1	B	Fractured zygoma
2	E	OM 0° and OM 30°
3	H	Left
4	L	Interpersonal trauma
5	P	Campbell

8.14 Facial Fractures (2)

1　A　Masseter

2　F　Gillies' hook

3　K　Infra-orbital

4　O　Cloudy

5　Q　Have you lost consciousness?

A fractured zygoma normally occurs as a result of interpersonal trauma, and as most people are right-handed, they tend to make contact with the left side of the face. The masseter inserts into the anterior two-thirds of the zygomatic arch, and the injury leads to trismus frequently. The infra-orbital nerve is commonly damaged temporarily in this fracture, and the antrum has a cloudy appearance. It is extremely important to ask if the patient has lost consciousness, as this is a sign of brain injury and the patient needs to be observed. The pupils need to be assessed to see if they are equal and reactive to light.

8.15 Bone Lesions

1　B　Osteomyelitis

2　E　Sequestrum

3　D　Involucrum

4　I　Moth-eaten

5　L　Mandible

Osteomyelitis is a spreading, progressive inflammation of the bone and bone marrow, more frequently affecting the mandible. It produces a moth-eaten appearance. There is evidence of the sequestrum (dead bone) and involucrum (newly formed bone).

8.16 Benign Tumours

1	C	Fibrous dysplasia
2	F	10-20 years
3	J	Maxilla
4	O	Posterior
5	P	Round

8.17 Radiological Diagnosis

1	A	Poorly defined
2	F	PET
3	I	Mixed radiopaque and radiolucent
4	K	Orange peel
5	M	Bucco-lingual

Fibrous dysplasia is considered to represent a developmental tumour-like lesion. 80% are monostotic. It tends to occur in the 10-20 years age group. It most commonly occurs in the posterior maxilla, but may spread to other bones. Radiographically, it is round and poorly defined, with the margins merging with adjacent bone. The lesion is initially radiolucent, but gradually becomes radiopaque to produce the typical orange peel or ground glass appearance. This results from the superimposition of many fine, poorly calcified bone trabeculae arranged in a disorganised fashion. The adjacent teeth are sometimes displaced, but rarely resorbed. There is bucco-lingual expansion, and as stated above, it spreads to adjacent bones.

8.18 Non-Odontogenic Cysts

1   C   Nasopalatine duct cyst

2   G   40-60 years

3   J   1%

4   M   Anterior maxilla

5   P   Smooth and well defined

Nasopalatine cysts develop from the epithelial remnants of the nasopalatine duct or incisive canal. They are most frequently detected in the 40-60 years age group. They are the most common non-odontogenic cysts and affect 1% of the population. They occur in the midline of the anterior maxilla. The size is variable, but usually greater than 6 mm. The shape is round or oval and monolocular, and the outline smooth and well defined. These cysts are radiolucent and rarely affect adjacent teeth.

8.19 Malignant Tumours (1)

1   B   Multiple myeloma

2   E   Male

3   H   Skull vault

4   M   40-60 years

5   O   African-Caribbean

8.20 Malignant Tumours (2)

1   A   Plasma cells

2   F   Pepper pot skull

3   H   Radiolucent

4   K   Monolocular

5   N   Bence Jones

Multiple myeloma is a lymphoreticular tumour of bone. Multifocal proliferation of the plasma cell series within the bone marrow results in overproduction of immunoglobulins. Multiple myeloma occurs mainly in middle-aged African-Caribbean men, and affects the skull vault and many other bones. It produces monolocular, but multifocal, round and punched-out lesions. This gives the skull the classic 'pepper pot' appearance.

8.21 Oral Tumours (5)

1   D   Complex odontome

2   C   Compound odontome

Odontomes are found in two forms:

1. Complex

2. Compound

It is important to be able to spot the difference. They are a favourite in paedodontic vivas.

8.22 More Cysts

1 C Radicular cyst

2 D Male

3 H Acquired via trauma

4 L Anterior maxilla

5 N Buccal

6 S 75%

7 T Rests of Malassez

8 W Monolocular

Radicular cysts are inflammatory cysts which develop from the rests of Malassez. They occur in the 20–50-year-old age group and account for 75% of all jaw cysts. They occur at the apex of non-vital teeth, particularly upper lateral and central incisors. They are usually between 1.5 cm and 3 cm in size. (If they are smaller they are indistinguishable from periapical granulomas.) The lesion is small, monolocular, round, smooth and well defined, and also uniformly radiolucent. The cyst expands buccally, occasionally displaces teeth and more rarely resorbs teeth.

8.23 Salivary Glands

1	D	Sjögren syndrome

2	E	Sialography

3	I	Parotid gland

4	M	Snow storm

5	P	Rheumatoid arthritis

Sjögren syndrome is an autoimmune condition found mainly in middle-aged women. It causes dry mouth, dry eyes and dry genitals. There is increased root caries and problems with taste. The definitive diagnosis is with a labial gland biopsy deep to muscle. Sialography and the presence of autoantibodies may help to confirm the diagnosis but are not definitive. Treatment is with pilocarpine and saliva substitutes.

8.24 Trauma (1)

1	C	Fractured orbital floor

2	F	OM

3	I	CT

4	N	Retrobulbar haemorrhage

5	P	Hanging drop

8.25 Trauma (2)

1	B	Enophthalmos
2	E	Diplopia
3	H	Interpersonal trauma
4	K	Retinal detachment
5	O	Do not blow your nose

A fractured orbital floor presents generally after interpersonal trauma – a blow to the face. The 'blow-out' fracture causes the herniation of the contents of the orbital floor into the maxillary sinus. Radiographically the contents of the floor give the 'hanging drop' sign. The medical emergency is retrobulbar haemorrhage – bleeding behind the eye can lead to blindness. This needs surgery within an hour to stop the bleeding and prevent a build-up of pressure, which causes the blindness. Patients should be advised not to blow their nose, as this may displace an undisplaced fracture.

8.26 Oral Tumours (6)

| 1 | A | Ameloblastoma |

| 2 | F | 35–50 years |

| 3 | H | Posterior mandible |

| 4 | M | Multilocular |

| 5 | P | Soap bubble |

Ameloblastoma is an aggressive non-metastasising tumour that originates from remnants of the odontogenic epithelium. It is the most common odontogenic tumour and occurs in adults around the age of 40. Ameloblastomas usually occur in the posterior mandible, and only in rare cases involve the maxilla. Radiographically they are multilocular with distinct septa that divide the lesion into compartments with large, apparently discrete areas centrally and smaller areas at the periphery. They have a soap bubble appearance. The outline is smooth and scalloped. Ameloblastomas are well defined and well corticated. The lesion is radiolucent with internal radiopaque septa. Adjacent teeth are displaced, loosened and resorbed. There is extensive expansion in all directions.

9
Restorative Dentistry and Materials

9.1 Theme: Anatomical Features associated with Complete Dentures
9.2 Theme: Constituents of Dental Toothpaste
9.3 Theme: Histological Zones in Enamel Caries
9.4 Theme: Optical Properties of Teeth and Restoration
9.5 Theme: Retention of Dental Restorations
9.6 Theme: Scope of Practice
9.7 Theme: Prosthodontic Components
9.8 Theme: Tooth Preparation Procedures
9.9 Theme: Tooth Surface Loss
9.10 Theme: Restorative Materials
9.11 Theme: Cavities
9.12 Theme: Signs of Different Types of Dental Pain
9.13 Theme: Differentiation of Symptoms
9.14 Theme: Occlusion (1)
9.15 Theme: Occlusion (2)
9.16 Theme: Occlusion (3)
9.17 Theme: Dental Materials (1)
9.18 Theme: Endodontics
9.19 Theme: Root Canal Treatment
9.20 Theme: Partial Dentures (1)
9.21 Theme: Dental Anatomy
9.22 Theme: Working Lengths
9.23 Theme: Partial Dentures (2)
9.24 Theme: Partial Dentures (3)
9.25 Theme: Immediate Complete Dentures
9.26 Theme: Complete Dentures
9.27 Theme: Dental Materials (2)
9.28 Theme: Dental Materials (3)
9.29 Theme: Dental Materials (4)
9.30 Theme: Impression Compounds

RESTORATIVE DENTISTRY AND MATERIALS

9.1 Theme: Anatomical Features associated with Complete Dentures

A   External oblique ridge
B   Fovea palatini
C   Genial tubercles
D   Incisive papillae
E   Hamular notch
F   Maxillary tuberosity
G   Mylohyoid ridge
H   Retromolar pad

For each of the following clinical descriptions, choose the most appropriate anatomical features associated with complete dentures from the list above. You may use each option once, more than once or not at all.

1   Two small pits or depressions in the posterior aspect of the palatal mucosa, one on each side of the midline, at or near the attachment of the soft palate to the hard palate.

2   An oblique ridge on the lingual surface of the mandible that extends from the level of the roots of the last molar teeth and that serves as a bony attachment for the mylohyoid muscles forming the floor of the mouth.

3   The most distal portion of the maxillary alveolar ridge.

4   A mass of tissue comprised of non-keratinized mucosa located posterior to the retromolar papilla and overlying loose glandular connective tissue.

5   The palpable notch formed by the junction of the maxilla and the pterygoid hamulus of the sphenoid bone.

9.2 Theme: Constituents of Dental Toothpaste

A   Alginate
B   Calcium phosphate
C   Glycerol
D   Potassium nitrate
E   Silica
F   Sodium benzoate
G   Sodium lauryl sulphate
H   Sodium monofluorophosphate
I   Triclosan
J   Xylitol

From the options above of the constituents of dental toothpaste, choose the correct function of the constituent in toothpaste from the list below. You may use each option once, more than once or not at all.

1. Acts as a detergent
2. Acts as a binder
3. Humectant
4. Abrasive
5. Preservative

9.3 Theme: Histological Zones in Enamel Caries

A   Body
B   Dark
C   Demineralisation
D   Destruction
E   Invasion
F   Sclerosis
G   Surface
H   Translucent

For each of the following statements, choose the correct option from the list above. Each option may be used once, more than once, or not at all

1. 1% demineralization has occurred.
2. 2–4% demineralization has occurred.
3. 5% or more demineralization has occurred.
4. Advancing edge of lesion.
5. The bulk of the lesion.

RESTORATIVE DENTISTRY AND MATERIALS

9.4 Theme: Optical Properties of Teeth and Restoration

A	Chroma	E	Opalescence
B	Fluorescence	F	Texture
C	Hue	G	Translucency
D	Metamerism	H	Value

From the option list above of factors affecting the optical properties of teeth, choose the most appropriate option which is having the major impact. You may use each option once, more than once or not at all.

1. A patient complains that her new crown is too dark.
2. A patient complains that his upper right lateral incisor crown is more yellow than his canine tooth.
3. A patient notices that the new crown she has just received is more opaque than the adjacent incisor, which has a bluish tinge to the incisal edge.
4. You have just fitted a new porcelain veneer, and it appears too shiny compared to the adjacent teeth.
5. A patient returns and informs you that his crown appeared another colour while at work, but in the dental surgery the colour appears satisfactory.

9.5 Theme: Retention of Dental Restorations

A	Buccal/lingual groove/slot
B	Chemical bonding
C	Dentine pin
D	Dovetail
E	Minimally taper
F	Post
G	Proximal grooves
H	Undercuts over the occlusal floor

From the list above of ways in which restorations may be retained, choose the most appropriate answer. You may use each option once, more than once or not at all.

1. Repairing a distal box of an amalgam restoration in a large MODB restored molar.
2. A de-coronated root filled central incisor.
3. A small buccal cervical lesion in dentine.
4. A premolar requiring a full gold crown.
5. Placing a small amalgam restoration in a proximal box of a premolar.

9.6 Theme: Scope of Practice

A Clinical dental technician
B Dental hygienist
C Dental nurse
D Dental technician
E Dental therapist
F Orthodontic therapist

For each of the following legally permitted duties for dental care professionals, choose the most appropriate role from the list above. You may use each option once, more than once or not at all.

1 Directly restore the secondary dentition.
2 Fit headgear.
3 Fit removable dentures.
4 Place orthodontic brackets.
5 Replace implant abutment.

9.7 Theme: Prosthodontic Components

A Abutment
B Clasp
C Movable joint
D Pontic
E Post-dam
F Reciprocal arm
G Rest
H Retainer
I Saddle

For each of the following descriptions, choose the most appropriate component(s) or feature(s) from the list above. You may use each option once, more than once or not at all.

1 That component of a cobalt-chromium removable partial denture which enables clasps to be functional. These units may also provide bracing.
2 That component of a fixed bridge which helps in breaking stresses through the span. Allows for differential movement across the bridge.
3 The term used to describe the tooth or teeth to which a bridge is attached.

9.8 Theme: Tooth Preparation Procedures

A   Cingulum rest preparation
B   Composite restorations
C   Full-coverage crown
D   Guide plane preparation
E   Partial-coverage cast restoration
F   Tilting cast

For each of the following descriptions, choose the most appropriate preparation or procedure from the list above. You may use each option once, more than once or not at all.

1. Presence of deep hard tissue undercut associated with the anterior maxilla.
2. Modification of an unfavourable survey line, prior to recording a master impression.
3. Capacity to provide additional support and in certain circumstances indirect retention.

9.9 Theme: Tooth Surface Loss

A   Abfraction
B   Abrasion
C   Attrition
D   Caries
E   Erosion
F   Iatrogenic
G   Traumatic

For each of the following descriptions, choose the most appropriate process from the list above. You may use each option once, more than once or not at all.

1. Tooth surface loss which results from repeated cyclical loading and unloading, resulting in cervical tissue loss.
2. Tooth surface loss during access preparation for endodontics, or following debonding of orthodontic brackets.
3. Tooth surface loss characterised by sensitivity when actively occurring. Characterised by affected areas being shiny and smooth. Advanced lesions may be represented by occlusal cupping. Amalgam restorations may be noted to be sitting higher and proud of the remaining tooth tissue.

9.10 Theme: Restorative Materials

A   Amalgam alloy
B   Ceramics
C   Direct composite
D   Direct gold (foil) alloy
E   Glass ionomer cement
F   Indirect composite
G   Indirect gold alloy
H   Resin ionomer
I   Zinc oxide/eugenol
J   Zinc oxide restorative material

For each of the following statements, choose the most appropriate material from the list above. You may use each option once, more than once or not at all.

1. Excellent aesthetics, brittle in thin section, can be difficult to bond to tooth, constructed indirectly, can cause significant wear of the opposing teeth if occlusion is not correct.

2. Known to have a eutectoidal phase diagram, and is available in high and low copper varieties. Can be used as a restorative material, as a core material or in situations where moisture contamination and isolation are a problem.

3. A material with good to excellent aesthetics. Commonly used to construct restorations which are provided for posterior teeth, and are bonded in place. Tend not to suffer from bulk polymerisation shrinkage and are easy to repair in the mouth.

9.11 Theme: Cavities

A   Class I
B   Class II
C   Class III
D   Class IV
E   Class V

For each of the following descriptions of a dental cavity, choose the most appropriate term from the list above. You may use each option once, more than once or not at all.

1. A cavity in pits and fissures of a premolar/molar.
2. A cavity in approximal surface(s) of a molar/premolar.
3. A cavity in approximal surface of incisor/canine not involving the incisal edge.
4. A cavity in approximal surface of incisor/canine involving the incisal edge.
5. A cavity in the cervical third or buccal or lingual surface of any tooth.

9.12 Theme: Signs of Different Types of Dental Pain

A   Acute periapical abscess
B   Cracked-tooth syndrome
C   Dentine hypersensitivity
D   Irreversible pulpitis
E   Lateral periodontal abscess
F   Reversible pulpitis

For each of the following problems, choose the most likely cause above. You may use each option once, more than once or not at all.

1. Tooth usually mobile with lateral tender to percussion (TTP) and associated localised or diffuse swelling of the adjacent periodontium.

2. The tooth is usually extruded with apical TTP. It may be associated with a localised or diffuse swelling. Radiographic changes show a widening of the periodontal ligament.

3. Very few signs, which may only be seen when biting on a cotton wool roll.

4. Diagnosis by elimination, and from using cold or hot to elicit symptoms.

5. Exaggerated response to pulp testing. Carious cavity or leaking restoration present.

6. Application of heat (eg warm gutta percha) elicits pain. Affected tooth may give low or absent response to pulp testing. A carious cavity/leaking restoration is present.

9.13 Theme: Differentiation of Symptoms

A   Acute periapical abscess
B   Cracked-tooth syndrome
C   Dentine hypersensitivity
D   Irreversible pulpitis
E   Lateral periodontal abscess
F   Reversible pulpitis

For each of the following scenarios, choose the most likely diagnosis from the list above. You may use each option once, more than once or not at all.

1 Spontaneous pain which may last for several hours, be worse at night and it is often pulsatile in nature. Pain is elicited by hot and cold at first but in later stages heat is more significant. Pain remains after the stimulus has been removed.

2 Pain is only elicited in response to a thermal, tactile or osmotic stimulus.

3 Sharp pain on biting – short duration.

4 Acute pain and tenderness often with an associated bad taste.

5 Severe pain which will disturb sleep. Tooth is exquisitely tender to touch.

6 Fleeting pain/sensitivity to hot, cold or sweet with immediate onset. Pain is usually sharp and may be difficult to locate. Quickly subsides after the removal of stimulus.

9.14 Theme: Occlusion (1)

A	Balanced occlusion	F	Group function
B	Canine-guided occlusion	G	Ideal occlusion
C	Centric stops	H	Interferences
D	Freeway space	I	Rest position
E	Functional occlusion		

For each of the following definitions, choose the most appropriate term from the list above. You may use each option once, more than once or not at all.

1. Anatomically perfect occlusion.

2. An occlusion that is free of interferences to smooth gliding movements of the mandible, with the absence of pathology.

3. Balancing the contacts in all excursions of the mandible to provide increased stability of complete/complete dentures, not applicable to natural dentition.

4. Multiple tooth contacts on working side during lateral excursions, but no contact on the non-working side.

5. During lateral excursions there is disclusion of all the teeth on the working side, except the canines.

9.15 Theme: Occlusion (2)

A	Centric occlusion
B	Centric relation
C	Hinge axis
D	Retruded arc of closure
E	Terminal hinge axis

For each of the following definitions, choose the most appropriate term from the list above. You may use each option once, more than once or not at all.

1. The axis of rotation of the condyles during the first few millimetres of mandibular opening.

2. The axis of rotation of the mandible when the condyles are in their most posterior, superior position in the glenoid fossa.

3. The arc of closure of the mandible with the condyles rotating about the terminal hinge axis.

4. Position of maximum interdigitation.

5. Position of the mandible where initial tooth contact occurs on the retruded arc of closure.

9.16 Theme: Occlusion (3)

A	Centric stops	E	Interferences
B	Deflective contacts	F	Non-supporting cusps
C	Freeway space	G	Occlusal vertical dimension
D	Functional cusps	H	Rest position

For each of the following definitions, choose the most appropriate term from the list above. You may use each option once, more than once or not at all.

1. Contacts which hinder smooth excursive movements of the mandible.
2. Relationship between the mandible and the maxilla in centric occlusion, ie face height.
3. Cusps that do not occlude with opposing teeth.
4. The habitual postural position of the mandible when the patient is relaxed with the condyles in a neutral position.
5. Cusps that occlude with the centric stops on the opposing tooth.
6. The difference between the rest and intercuspal position.
7. The points on the occlusal surface which meet with the opposing tooth in centric occlusion.
8. Cause the deflection of the mandible from the natural path of closure.

9.17 Theme: Dental Materials (1)

A	Canal irrigant
B	Direct pulp cap
C	Material used to aid apexification
D	Material used to aid passage through canal narrowing
E	Steroid/antibiotic paste

For each of the following materials, choose the most appropriate use from the list above. You may use each option once, more than once or not at all.

1. EDTA
2. Non-setting calcium hydroxide
3. Setting calcium hydroxide
4. Ledermix
5. Sodium hypochlorite

9.18 Theme: Endodontics

A   Anticurvature filing
B   Balanced-force technique
C   Stepback technique
D   Stepdown technique
E   Standardised technique

For each of the following definitions of endodontic preparatory techniques, choose the most appropriate term from the list above. You may use each option once, more than once or not at all.

1. This technique prepares the coronal part of the canal before the apical part. A very popular method of preparation with rotary instruments.
2. A method devised to prevent strip perforations on the inner walls of curved root canals. It involves a filing ratio of 3:1 outer wall: inner wall.
3. This technique uses reamers or K-files with a rotary action to prepare the apical part of the canal to a round cross-section.
4. The apical part of the canal is prepared first and the canal is flared from the apex to crown.
5. A complex technique involving the use of blunt-tipped files with an anticlockwise rotation while applying an apically directed force.

9.19 Theme: Root Canal Treatment

A   Coated carriers
B   Cold lateral condensation
C   Thermoplasticised injectable gutta percha
D   Vertical condensation
E   Warm lateral condensation

For each of the following descriptions, choose the most appropriate term from the list above. You may use each option once, more than once or not at all.

1. Cores of titanium or plastic that are coated with gutta percha. They are heated in an oven and pushed into a canal at the correct length.
2. A master apical cone is placed in the canal and accessory cones are obturated around it.
3. A master apical cone is placed in the canal and accessory cones are placed around it and they are then compacted with a warm spreader.
4. A commercial machine extrudes heated gutta percha into the canal.
5. Gutta percha is warmed using a heated instrument and packed vertically.

9.20 Theme: Partial Dentures (1)

A   Abutment
B   Bridge
C   Connector
D   Pontic
E   Resistance
F   Retainer
G   Retention
H   Saddle
I   Support
J   Unit

For each of the following descriptions, choose the most appropriate term from the list above. You may use each option once, more than once or not at all.

1   A tooth which provides attachment for a bridge.
2   The artificial tooth suspended from abutments.
3   The component that is cemented to the abutments to provide retention of the prosthesis.
4   The area of edentulous ridge.
5   Prevents removal of the restoration along the path of insertion or along axis of the preparation.
6   Prevents dislodgement of the restoration by forces directed in an apical or oblique direction and prevents movement of the restoration under occlusal forces.
7   The ability of the abutment teeth to maintain the load on the restoration.

9.21 Theme: Dental Anatomy

A 0
B 1
C 2
D 3
E 4

For each of the following teeth, choose the most appropriate number of root canals from the list above. You may use each option once, more than once or not at all.

1 Lower first permanent molar
2 Upper first permanent molar
3 Upper second permanent premolar
4 Lower first permanent premolar
5 Lower second permanent molar

9.22 Theme: Working Lengths

A 17 mm
B 18 mm
C 19 mm
D 19.5 mm
E 20 mm
F 21 mm
G 22 mm
H 23 mm
I 24 mm
J 25 mm

For each of the following teeth, choose the most appropriate average working length from the list above. You may use each option once, more than once or not at all.

1 Maxillary central incisor
2 Mandibular central incisor
3 Maxillary canine
4 Mandibular canine
5 Maxillary premolar
6 Mandibular premolar
7 Maxillary first permanent molar
8 Mandibular first permanent molar

9.23 Theme: Partial Dentures (2)

A   Kennedy Class I
B   Kennedy Class II
C   Kennedy Class III
D   Kennedy Class IV
E   Craddock Class I
F   Craddock Class II
G   Craddock Class III

For each of the following denture designs, choose the most appropriate classification from the list above. You may use each option once, more than once or not at all.

1   Unilateral bounded saddle
2   Unilateral free end saddle
3   Tooth-borne denture
4   Mucosa- and tooth-borne denture
5   Anterior bounded saddle only

9.24 Theme: Partial Dentures (3)

A   First stage
B   Second stage
C   Third stage
D   Fourth stage
E   Fifth stage
F   Sixth stage

For each of the following steps of partial denture design, choose the most appropriate stage in the design from the list above. You may use each option once, more than once or not at all.

1   Plan support
2   Obtain retention
3   Surveying
4   Assess bracing
5   Choose connector
6   Outline saddles

9.25 Theme: Immediate Complete Dentures

A	First stage
B	Second stage
C	Third stage
D	Fourth stage
E	Fifth stage
F	Sixth stage
G	Seventh stage

For each of the following steps in immediate denture preparation, choose the most appropriate stage in the preparation from the list above. You may use each option once, more than once or not at all.

1. Secondary impressions
2. Finish
3. Extraction
4. Assessment
5. Primary impressions
6. Record occlusion
7. Try-in

9.26 Theme: Complete Dentures

A	Alteration of palatal contour, incorrect overjet and overbite
B	Incisors too far back palatally
C	Lack of retention
D	Palatal vault too high behind the incisors
E	Palate too thick

For each of the following problems with complete dentures, choose the most likely cause from the list above. You may use each option once, more than once or not at all.

1. Difficulty with saying the letters f and v
2. Difficulty with saying the letters d, s and t
3. When trying to say the letter s, it becomes 'the'
4. Whistling
5. Clicking teeth

9.27 Theme: Dental Materials (2)

A Elastic limit
B Elastic modulus
C Resilience
D Stiffness
E Strain
F Stress
G Toughness

For each of the following definitions, choose the most appropriate term from the list above. You may use each option once, more than once or not at all.

1. The change in size of a material that occurs in response to a force. It is calculated by dividing the change in length by the original length.

2. A measure of the rigidity of a material defined by the ratio of stress to strain (below the elastic limit).

3. The amount of energy absorbed up to the point of fracture. It is a function of the resilience of the material and its ability to undergo plastic deformation rather than fracture.

4. The stress beyond which a material is permanently deformed when a force is applied.

5. The energy absorbed by a material undergoing elastic deformation up to its elastic limit.

6. The internal force set up in reaction to, and opposite to, the applied force. Can be classified according to the direction of the force – tensile (stretching), compressive or shear.

7. This gives an indication of how easy it is to bend a material without causing a permanent deformation or fracture.

9.28 Theme: Dental Materials (3)

A	Coefficient of thermal expansion	E	Thermal conductivity
B	Creep	F	Thermal diffusivity
C	Fatigue	G	Wear
D	Hardness	H	Wettability

For each of the following statements, choose the most appropriate term from the list above. You may use each option once, more than once or not at all.

1. The slow plastic deformation that occurs with application of force over time.
2. The ability of a material to transmit heat.
3. The fractional increase in length for each degree of temperature rise.
4. The resistance to penetration.
5. The abrasion resistance of a substance.
6. The rate at which temperature changes spread through a material.
7. The ability of one material to flow across the surface of another.
8. When cyclic forces are applied, a crack may nucleate and grow by small increments each time the force is applied.

9.29 Theme: Dental Materials (4)

A	Copper
B	Palladium
C	Platinum
D	Silver
E	Zinc

For each of the following benefits of adding elements to gold alloys, choose the most appropriate element the list above. You may use each option once, more than once or not at all.

1. Increased tarnish resistance.
2. Scavenger, prevents oxidation of other metals during melting and casting.
3. Increased strength and hardness.
4. Decreased density and melting point.
5. Increased density and melting point.
6. Increased corrosion.
7. Increased porosity.

9.30 Theme: Impression Compounds

A Addition-cured silicone
B Condensation-cured silicone
C Impression compound
D Irreversible hydrocolloid (alginate)
E Polyether
F Polysulphide
G Reversible hydrocolloid
H Zinc oxide paste

For each of the following descriptions of impression materials, choose the correct name from the list above. You may use each option once, more than once or not at all.

1 Available in a sheet form for recording preliminary impressions. This material is softened in a water bath at 55–60°C and used in a stock tray to record edentulous ridges.

2 A popular material because it uses a single mix and a stock tray (and smells of gin and tonic). The set material is stiff and removal can be stressful in cases with deep undercuts or advanced periodontitis. Absorbs water, and should not be stored with alginate impressions.

3 An accurate hydrocolloid material, but is liable to tearing. Requires the purchase of a water bath.

4 This is a very cheap elastomer, prone to shrinkage and should be cast immediately.

5 This is a very stable silicone elastomer. It allows impressions to be cast later, and even posted to the laboratory. However, casting within 1 hour is contraindicated, and latex gloves can retard setting.

6 This elastomer wets the preparation well, but is messy to handle. It is useful when a long working time is required. Should be used with a special tray and although stable, cast within 24 hours.

7 This is dispensed and mixed to give an even colour. It is used for recording edentulous ridges in a special tray or the patient's existing dentures, but is contraindicated in undercuts.

8 The setting reaction is a double decomposition reaction involving calcium sulphate. Popular because it is cheap and can be used in a stock tray. Not sufficiently accurate for crown and bridge work.

9.1 Anatomical Features associated with Complete Dentures

1	B	Fovea palatini
2	G	Mylohyoid ridge
3	F	Maxillary tuberosity
4	H	Retromolar pad
5	E	Hamular notch

The buccal shelf is bordered externally by the external oblique line and internally by the slope of the residual ridge. This region is a primary stress bearing area in the mandibular arch.

Incisive papilla is a pad of fibrous connective tissue overlying the orifice of the nasopalatine canal; the central incisors are normally set up to 10 mm anterior to the incisive papilla.

The fovea palatine are located close to the vibrating line where the posterior palatal extension of the maxillary denture should be located.

The genial tubercles or **mental spines**; rounded elevations (usually two pairs) clustered around the midline on the lingual surface of the lower portion of the mandibular symphysis. These tubercles serve as attachments for the genioglossus and geniohyoid muscles and limit the anterior labial flange of the mandibular denture.

The hamular notch is critical to the design of the maxillary denture. Improper molding of this area could lead to soreness and loss of retention particularly in an anterio-posterior direction.

The maxillary tuberosities can aid retention of the maxillary denture but if they are over developed or have undercuts present they may hinder retention and may require surgical correction.

The mylohyoid ridge is a border limitation on the lingual margin of a mandibular flange.

With the retromolar pad the bone beneath does not resorb secondary to the pressure associated with denture use. It is one of the primary support areas.

9.2 Constituents of Dental Toothpaste

1 G Sodium lauryl sulphate

2 A Alginate

3 C Glycerol

4 E Silica

5 F Sodium benzoate

Calcium phosphate and sodium monofluorophosphate help to remineralise early carious lesions. Potassium nitrate may be added as a desensitising agent along with potassium chloride or potassium oxalate. Triclosan is antibacterial and xylitol is a sweetner.

9.3 Histological Zones in Enamel Caries

1 G Surface

2 B Dark

3 A Body

4 H Translucent

5 A Body

The histological zones for enamel caries from the surface to the advancing edge are:

- Surface
- Body
- Dark
- Translucent

The other zones mentioned - namely, destruction, invasion (sometimes referred to as zone of bacterial penetration), demineralization and sclerosis - occur in dentinal caries from the outermost to innermost.

9.4 Optical Properties of Teeth and Restoration

1 H Value

2 A Chroma

3 G Translucency

4 F Texture

5 D Metamerism

The value is the gray scale from white to black. High value means very white and low value is very dark or black. If a crown is too dark, the value has been too low.

Chroma is the intensity of colour, while hue is the actual colour. For example, if one drop of yellow is added to a beaker of water and 10 drops of yellow are added to another similar-sized beaker of water, both beakers would have the same hue but the second beaker would have more chroma (intensity).

Translucency occurs in younger teeth and frequently gives a bluish tinge to the incisal edge of teeth. Crowns and veneers can have translucent porcelain, but practitioners frequently do not mention translucency on the crown prescriptions to technicians. Opalescence may also give a blue/grey/violet appearance, but usually it extends over a greater area of the tooth.

Surface texture is essential for breaking up the reflected light. If too little surface texture is added, the restoration will appear shiny and possibly false.

Metamerism is when objects appear to be a different colour in different spectral light. Hence there can be differences between natural and fluorescent light. It is important to ask the individual in what environment they will spend most of their time and try to match the restoration in a similar light source.

9.5 Retention of Dental Restorations

1 D Dovetail

2 F Post

3 B Chemical bonding

4 E Minimally taper

5 G Proximal grooves

A dovetail or key-way cut into a large amalgam is one way to retain a proximal box. In small restorations proximal grooves may be sufficient.

When root-filled incisors have little coronal tissue, left posts are required to retain the core restoration before placing a crown.

Small buccal cervical restorations usually involve dentine and are restored with glass ionomer cements, which chemically bond to the tooth.

Crown restorations usually rely on minimal taper in order to retain the crown. The cement lute used usually is a 'space' filler between the tooth and the restoration. Chemically bonding cements may be indicated when the geometry of the preparation means that the taper was not minimal (below 10 degrees). However, if the tooth is of normal height, even tapers of up to 20 degrees have been found to be clinically acceptable.

It is now debatable whether amalgam should be used in small proximal boxes, as composites would be less destructive for retention. When amalgam is used, the proximal grooves add retention. Composites are retained by etching the enamel; this causes differential dissolution of the enamel surface, creating micro-porosities which the resin can micro-mechanically retain to.

Dentine pins were used to help retain large amalgam restorations. They are now rarely used due to the risk of pulpal exposure and dentine fractures.

364 RESTORATIVE DENTISTRY AND MATERIALS

9.6 Scope of Practice

| 1 | E | Dental therapist |

| 2 | F | Orthodontic therapist |

| 3 | A | Clinical dental technician |

| 4 | F | Orthodontic therapist |

| 5 | A | Clinical dental technician |

Only dental therapists are allowed to directly restore the secondary dentition. Orthodontic therapists are allowed to fit orthodontic headgear and brackets under the prescription of a dentist. Clinical dental technicians may fit removable dentures and replace implant abutments for removable prostheses under the prescription of a dentist.

The General Dental Council have published guidance for dental care professionals, outlining the skills and abilities each registrant group should have, and listing all their legally-permitted duties. See 'Scope of Practice', effective from 30 Sept 2013.

9.7 Theme: Prosthodontic Components

| 1 | F | Reciprocal arm |

This component of a removable partial denture reciprocates the action of the clasp. This allows the clasp to be functional. Reciprocal arms are also capable of providing bracing of the denture, and prevent unfavourable lateral displacement.

| 2 | C | Movable joint |

This is a component present between a pontic and an abutment (usually mesial), and allows for small vertical movements between the two. The design helps to reduce stress within the bridge.

| 3 | A | Abutment |

The abutment is the tooth or teeth to which a bridge is attached. The retainer is that part of a bridge which is attached to the abutment teeth.

9.8 Tooth Preparation Procedures

1 F Tilting cast

Deep hard tissue undercuts can either by eliminated or utilised. The cast can be tilted on the surveyor in order to either utilise or eliminate the undercut.

2 B Composite restorations

This technique can be used to either add composite to the tooth, or remove tissue. These procedures can be used in order to raise or lower survey lines, such that the dentist is able to provide a denture design with the clasps and reciprocal arms in desirable positions.

3 A Cingulum rest preparation

Rest seats are used to provide support. These may also provide indirect retention when suitably located.

9.9 Tooth Surface Loss

1 A Abfraction

2 F Iatrogenic

Tooth tissue may be lost secondary to dental procedures.

3 E Erosion

Acid dissolution of the tooth surfaces results in shiny smooth tooth surfaces. The location is dependent upon the source of the acid. Times of active dissolution can be associated with periods of sensitivity and possibly pain. Amalgam restorations often sit proud of the affected enamel surface, as both materials show differing extents of acid dissolution.

9.10 Restorative Materials

1 B Ceramics

Ceramic materials can offer exceptional aesthetics. Restorations made of this material are laboratory-made, or at the chairside by means of computer-aided design and manufacture. These materials are strong in bulk, but are prone to chipping and in heavy occlusions can cause significant wear of the opposing dentition. Due to their inert nature at room and mouth temperature, they can be challenging to bond to tooth tissue.

2 A Amalgam alloy

Dental amalgam is an alloy obtained from mixing silver, tin, zinc, copper and mercury. Older preparations were available with a lower quantity of copper. Newer preparations are available as high copper varieties. These high copper varieties have the advantage of providing more rapid set, and thus may be used to construct a core and be prepared for a crown in one visit. In addition to this, the high copper varieties of amalgam are said to notably reduce or eliminate the soft, corrosive, $\gamma2$ phase, improving the material's strength and durability. Dental amalgam is known as a eutectic alloy; its melting point is lower than that of any of the constituent metals within it.

3 F Indirect composite

Indirect composites are constructed in the laboratory. They are often used to provide medium-to-large-sized aesthetic restorations, often of the inlay type and sometimes the onlay type. Like their 'direct-type' counterpart, they are constructed from resin with glass filler particles. They offer a good tooth-coloured restorative option, but tend to minimise the effect of the polymerisation shrinkage by being cured under high temperatures and pressures, in a light cure box in a laboratory. Unlike porcelains, which can be difficult to repair acceptably, direct chairside composites can be used to repair indirect composite restorations also.

RESTORATIVE DENTISTRY AND MATERIALS

9.11 Cavities

1   A   Class I

2   B   Class II

3   C   Class III

4   D   Class IV

5   E   Class V

Thorough knowledge of the classification and description of cavities is important.

9.12 Signs of Different Types of Dental Pain

1   E   Lateral periodontal abscess

2   A   Acute periapical abscess

3   B   Cracked-tooth syndrome

4   C   Dentine hypersensitivity

5   D   Irreversible pulpitis

6   F   Reversible pulpitis

Apical periodontal abscess and lateral periodontal abscess can be differentiated in that in a lateral periodontal abscess the tooth is usually vital and a periodontal pocket is present. In an apical periodontal abscess the tooth is non-vital. Cracked-tooth syndrome is difficult to diagnose until you remove the restoration. Dentine hypersensitivity is diagnosed by elimination, as there are no physical signs.

9.13 Differentiation of Symptoms

1. D Irreversible pulpitis
2. C Dentine hypersensitivity
3. B Cracked-tooth syndrome
4. E Lateral periodontal abscess
5. A Acute periapical abscess
6. F Reversible pulpitis

As an old saying goes 'The patient tells you the diagnosis if you listen long enough'. If you ask the correct questions, you can elicit enough information to help you try to differentiate where, and what type of problem the patient has. Whether pulpitis is irreversible or reversible can be difficult to differentiate, but they are often described in exam questions.

9.14 Occlusion (1)

1. G Ideal occlusion
2. E Functional occlusion
3. A Balanced occlusion
4. F Group function
5. B Canine-guided occlusion

Restorative consultants get very excited by occlusion, and it is a subject which if known well can save a lot of time in practice. The definitions are a part of this subject which can be easily examined.

RESTORATIVE DENTISTRY AND MATERIALS

9.15 Occlusion (2)

1 C Hinge axis

2 E Terminal hinge axis

3 D Retruded arc of closure

4 A Centric occlusion

5 B Centric relation

9.16 Occlusion (3)

1 E Interferences

2 G Occlusal vertical dimension

3 F Non-supporting cusps

4 H Rest position

5 D Functional cusps

6 C Freeway space

7 A Centric stops

8 B Deflective contacts

It is important to know the jargon when learning about restorative dentistry, as there is so much of it! But it enables you to understand occlusion more easily, which is probably the most important and difficult subject.

9.17 Dental Materials (1)

1. D Material used to aid passage through canal narrowing

2. C Material used to aid apexification

3. B Direct pulp cap

4. E Steroid/antibiotic paste

5. A Canal irrigant

Using the correct materials in endodontic situations is important. Hypochlorite is the most effective canal irrigant, as it has a powerful antibacterial action. It should be used with great care and good suction, as soft tissues can be damaged very easily with this. Setting calcium hydroxide (Dycal) is used as a material for direct pulp capping in a small exposure, and as a liner in other cases where there is no exposure. EDTA is a useful material that aids endodontic instrumentation in narrowed canals. Ledermix is not available in some countries; however, it is a useful material if the pulp is inflamed and cannot be extirpated. Ledermix often enables extirpation at the next visit. Non-setting calcium hydroxide is used to enable apexification, usually in traumatised immature permanent teeth.

9.18 Endodontics

1 D Stepdown technique

2 A Anticurvature filing

3 E Standardised technique

4 C Stepback technique

5 B Balanced-force technique

The most important manual technique is the stepback technique. This is extremely popular for undergraduates. Rotary instruments are very popular in practice and they are generally used for the stepdown technique. Rotary instruments have an advantage in that they prepare the canal faster and produce a preparation that fits a single piece of gutta percha with a perfect seal. However, their use is associated with greater incidence of perforation and instrument fracture.

9.19 Root Canal Treatment

1 A Coated carriers

2 B Cold lateral condensation

3 E Warm lateral condensation

4 C Thermoplasticised injectable gutta percha

5 D Vertical condensation

Cold lateral condensation is the most common method used by an undergraduate; however, students need to be aware of different methods which are used in practice. Most authorities but not all recommend thermal methods. This is because the filling material can enter into lateral canals and is more malleable in curved canals, producing a better filling result. However, there are differences in opinion with regard to what is the most important part of endodontic treatment. Experts debate and disagree on whether coronal seal or apical seal or cleaning of the canal is the most important part of treatment. Probably all parts are important in producing a symptom-free tooth.

9.20 Partial Dentures (1)

1 A Abutment

2 D Pontic

3 F Retainer

4 H Saddle

5 G Retention

6 E Resistance

7 I Support

In the discussion of clinical cases during finals, students are frequently asked about bridges and dentures. A good understanding of resistance, support and retention is very important.

9.21 Dental Anatomy

1 D 3

2 D 3

3 C 2

4 B 1

5 D 3

Remember, although the above is true, 25% of upper second premolars have more than one canal. Upper permanent molars should be treated as having four canals (2 mesiobuccal; 1 palatal; 1 distobuccal), until a second mesiobuccal canal cannot be found. 40% of lower incisors have 2 canals, but separate foramina are seen only in 1%.

9.22 Working Lengths

1 F 21 mm

2 E 20 mm

3 J 25 mm

4 I 24 mm

5 C 19 mm

6 E 20 mm

7 C 19 mm

8 D 19.5 mm

It is important to know what to expect in terms of working length, so that the tactile sensation when you are instrumenting a canal can be matched with the expected length. This can help you to decide whether you are close to the apex of a tooth or too short or too long.

The following table shows the expected working lengths of permanent teeth in millimetres.

	1	2	3	4/5	6	7
Maxilla	21	20	25	19	19	18.5
Mandible	20	19.5	24	20	19.5	18.5

9.23 Partial Dentures (2)

1 C Kennedy Class III

2 B Kennedy Class II

3 F Craddock Class II

4 G Craddock Class III

5 D Kennedy Class IV

The Kennedy Classification of dentures is based on the pattern of tooth loss:

I – Bilateral free end saddles
II – Unilateral free end saddle
III – Unilateral bounded saddle
IV – Anterior bounded saddle, only

Craddock describes the denture type:

I – Mucosa-borne
II – Tooth-borne
III – Mucosa- and tooth-borne

9.24 Partial Dentures (3)

1	C	Third stage
2	D	Fourth stage
3	A	First stage
4	E	Fifth stage
5	F	Sixth stage
6	B	Second stage

The correct order of steps in partial denture design is:

1 – surveying
2 – outline saddles
3 – plan support
4 – obtain retention
5 – assess bracing required
6 – choose connector.

Always reassess afterwards.

9.25 Immediate Complete Dentures

1	C	Third stage
2	G	Seventh stage
3	F	Sixth stage
4	A	First stage
5	B	Second stage
6	D	Fourth stage
7	E	Fifth stage

The clinical procedure is as follows. At assessment the number of teeth to be extracted should be decided, and the patient should be warned about bone resorption and the need for relining. Primary and secondary impressions should follow this. The occlusion should be recorded on the posterior teeth if there are sufficient remaining, or wax blocks should be used if this is not possible. The try-in is limited, as only those teeth already missing can be involved in this stage. Extraction should be performed as atraumatically as possible. The patient should be reviewed after 24 hours and then after 1 week.

RESTORATIVE DENTISTRY AND MATERIALS

9.26 Complete Dentures

1 B Incisors too far back palatally

2 A Alteration of palatal contour, incorrect overjet and overbite

3 E Palate too thick

4 D Palatal vault too high behind the incisors

5 C Lack of retention

Some denture problems can be sorted easily, and the above question covers these common problems. However, some patients with dentures can be difficult to treat. If a patient comes in with a bag of dentures, complaining that none of the dentures they possess are any good, it may be best to suggest they try a different dentist.

9.27 Dental Materials (2)

1 E Strain

2 B Elastic modulus

3 G Toughness

4 A Elastic limit

5 C Resilience

6 F Stress

7 D Stiffness

Dental materials is a well-hated subject because of its definitions and confusing physics. If you know the definitions and try to understand them, then the rest of it becomes a lot easier.

9.28 Dental Materials (3)

ANSWERS

1 B Creep

2 E Thermal conductivity

3 A Coefficient of thermal expansion

4 D Hardness

5 G Wear

6 F Thermal diffusivity

7 H Wettability

8 C Fatigue

Dental materials is a subject that rarely grabs the imagination of the dental student. The above question describes some of the jargon which is associated with dentine-bonding agents and crown materials.

9.29 Dental Materials (4)

1 B Palladium

2 E Zinc

3 A Copper

4 A Copper

5 D Silver

6 C Platinum

7 D Silver

Copper decreases density and melting point and increases strength and hardness, but it has the disadvantage of decreased corrosion resistance. Silver increases the hardness and strength, but its disadvantage is that it increases tarnishing and porosity. Platinum and palladium are similar in that they increase the tarnish resistance but they also increase the melting point and decrease the corrosion resistance. Zinc and sometimes indium are scavengers which prevent the oxidation of other metals.

9.30 Impression Compounds

1 C Impression compound

2 E Polyether

3 G Reversible hydrocolloid

4 B Condensation-cured silicone

5 A Addition-cured silicone

6 F Polysulphide

7 H Zinc oxide paste

8 D Irreversible hydrocolloid (alginate)

Impression materials are commonly used in dentistry. A great deal of knowledge about these materials creates a good impression!

Index

abdominal distension 2.20
abdominal masses 2.16
abdominal pain 2.24
abducens nerve (CNVI) 3.1, 4.2
abscesses
    lateral periodontal 6.13
    pain 9.12, 9.13
abutments 9.7, 9.20
ACE inhibitors 3.7, 7.1
aciclovir 6.19
acid erosion 9.9
acidogenic theory 4.9
acromegaly 2.11, 2.31, 3.24
acute necrotising ulcerative gingivitis (ANUG) 3.4, 3.5, 6.8, 6.10
Addison's disease 2.11, 3.14, 3.24
adenocarcinoma 5.11
adverse drug reactions 1.31, 3.7, 6.14, 7.4, 7.7–7.8, 7.15, 7.21
AIDS/HIV 2.2
alcohol abuse 2.18, 7.6, 7.21
alfa blockers 7.1, 7.15
alkaline phosphatase 2.36, 3.28, 4.25
alveolar osteitis 5.30
Alzheimer's disease 7.6
amalgam 9.5, 9.10
ameloblastic fibroma 4.21, 5.26

ameloblastoma 4.12, 4.21, 5.26, 8.4, 8.26
amelogenesis imperfecta 1.31
amoebic dysentery 2.28
amylase 2.36
anaemia 2.6, 2.27
anaesthetics 5.3
analgesics 5.31, 7.3
    side effects 7.7, 7.8
anatomy 1.24, 5.4, 5.27, 5.33, 9.1
    cephalometrics 1.14–1.15, 1.23
    dental 9.21, 9.22
aneurysmal bone cyst 4.20, 8.4
angina 2.22, 7.11
ankylosing spondylitis 2.15
anorexia nervosa 2.1
antibiotics 5.31, 6.3, 6.24, 7.14, 7.29
    side-effects 1.31, 6.14, 7.7
anticoagulants 5.6, 7.11, 7.15
antihypertensives 3.7, 6.14, 7.1, 7.7, 7.11, 7.12
antimalarials 3.7
ANUG 3.4, 3.5, 6.8, 6.10
aortic aneurysm 2.16, 2.22
aortic regurgitation 2.9
aortic stenosis 2.9
aphthous ulcers 3.5, 3.21–3.22
Arestin 6.3
arrhythmias 2.9, 7.28

arthritis 7.27
articaine 5.3
articular eminence 5.33
ascites 2.20
aspirin 7.9, 7.11, 7.12
asthma 1.28, 2.14, 2.29, 7.16, 7.18
atenolol 7.11, 7.12
atrial fibrillation 2.9, 7.28
Atridox 6.3
autoimmune disease 4.1
    SLE 2.10, 2.12, 2.19, 3.8

back pain 2.15
bacterial infections 2.28, 2.30, 2.32, 2.35
    Gram stains 6.20
    oral 4.9, 6.6–6.7
    see also specific diseases
basic periodontal examination (BPE) 6.9, 6.15, 6.25
Bass tooth-brushing technique 1.6, 1.22
behaviour management 1.12
Behçet syndrome 3.26
Bell's palsy 4.2, 4.3
beta blockers 7.1, 7.7, 7.11, 7.12
biliary colic 2.24
blistering disorders 3.9, 3.10, 4.4
bone lesions 2.15, 3.28, 4.20, 4.25, 8.15
brainstem death 2.23

INDEX

breathing difficulties 2.5, 2.29
bridges 9.7, 9.20, 9.23, 9.24
Brown's tumour 5.23, 8.4
bucket-handle fracture 5.21
bulimia 2.1
bupivacaine 5.3
burning mouth syndrome 3.25

caecal carcinoma 2.16
calcification dates 1.26
calcifying epithelial odontogenic tumour 4.21, 5.26
calcifying odontogenic cyst 4.20
calcium-channel blockers 3.7, 6.14
calcium hydroxide 9.17
calculus 6.7
　salivary 3.3, 5.11
cancer
　death rates 2.3
　metastatic 2.15, 2.18
　multiple myeloma 2.10, 4.22, 8.19–8.20
　oral 5.17, 5.30
　other sites 2.13, 2.19, 2.20
Candida infections 2.2, 3.5, 4.8
captopril 3.7
carbamazepine 3.16
carbimazole 7.4
cardiovascular disease 2.7, 2.9, 2.22, 7.11, 7.12
caries 1.4, 1.25, 4.9–4.11, 9.3
cauda equina syndrome 2.15
cavernous sinus thrombosis 5.1
cavity classification 9.11
cellulitis 2.33
cementoma 4.21, 8.9–8.10
cephalometrics 1.14–1.15, 1.23
ceramic materials 9.10
cerebrospinal fluid leakage 5.1
cerebrovascular disease 2.21, 2.23
cervical spinal nerves 4.3, 5.9
cervical sympathetic chain 4.3
chancre 3.12, 4.23
Charter's tooth-brushing technique 1.6
Chediak–Higashi syndrome 6.5, 6.8
cherubism 8.4, 8.12
chest pain 2.22

child dental health 1.1–1.31
　congenital conditions 4.23, 5.7, 5.24
　periodontitis 6.11–6.12
child development 1.1
childhood illnesses 1.2, 1.28, 2.5
chisels 6.26
cholera 2.28
chromosomal abnormalities 1.3
　see also Down syndrome; Turner syndrome
chronic obstructive pulmonary disease (COPD) 7.16, 7.18
ciclosporin 6.14
cingulum rests 9.8
circumvallate papillae 5.4
cleidocranial dysostosis 1.31
clinical trials 7.26
clozapine 7.4
clubbing 2.26
cluster headache 3.2
co-amoxiclav 7.7
co-dydramol 7.3
codeine 7.8, 7.21
collapse 2.25
composite restorations 9.8, 9.10
concussion (tooth) 1.5
confusion 7.6
congestive cardiac failure 2.5, 2.9, 2.14, 2.18, 2.25, 2.33
consciousness, loss of 2.21, 8.14
Corsodyl 6.24
corticosteroids 3.14, 7.4
Coxsackie A virus 3.6
CPITN-C probes 6.17
cracked-tooth syndrome 9.12, 9.13
Craddock classification 9.23
cranial nerves 3.1, 4.2, 5.9, 5.10
　trigeminal neuralgia 3.2, 3.16
Crohn's disease 4.8
Cross syndrome 6.1
croup 2.5
crown fracture 1.5
crown restoration 9.4, 9.5
curettage 6.16
curettes 6.2, 6.26
Cushing disease 2.31
Cushing syndrome 2.11, 3.24
cystic hygroma 5.7

cysts
　non-odontogenic 3.3, 4.20, 5.7, 5.23, 8.4, 8.18
　odontogenic 4.14–4.19, 8.4, 8.5–8.8, 8.22
cytomegalovirus 2.2, 2.30, 2.35, 3.13, 5.14

debris index 6.25
deciduous teeth
　eruption 1.7, 1.9
　treatment 1.25
deep vein thrombosis 2.33
dementia 7.6
dens in dente 1.19
dental caries 1.4, 1.25, 4.9–4.11, 9.3
dental professionals 9.6
dentigerous cyst 4.16–4.17, 8.7–8.8
dentine hypersensitivity 9.12, 9.13
Dentomycin 6.24
dentures
　complete 9.1, 9.25–9.26
　partial 9.7, 9.20, 9.23–9.24
dependent oedema 2.33
depression 2.27
dermatomyositis polymyositis 2.12
dermoid cyst 3.3, 5.23
diabetes insipidus 2.31
diabetes mellitus 4.1, 6.23
　complications 2.17
　diagnosis 2.10, 2.11, 2.13, 3.24
　treatment 7.10, 7.13
diagnostic tests 2.36
diamorphine 7.3
diarrhoea 2.28
diclofenac 7.3
digoxin 7.15
diplopia 5.22, 8.25
discoloured teeth 1.31
diuretics 7.1, 7.9
Down syndrome 1.3, 3.27, 6.4, 6.5, 6.18
doxazosin 7.15
drugs of abuse 7.22
drugs, pharmaceutical *see* pharmacology
dry mouth 3.15
duodenal ulcer 2.24

eating disorders 2.1
ectodermal dysplasia 1.31

INDEX

eczema 1.28
EDTA 9.17
Edward syndrome 1.3
Ehlers-Danlos syndrome 3.26, 4.6, 6.4
electrocardiography 2.7
Elyzol 6.3, 6.24
emergencies
   cardiovascular 7.12
   in the dental chair 5.12
   trauma 5.22, 5.32, 8.25
endocrine disease 2.11, 2.31, 3.14, 3.24
endodontics 9.18–9.19
enophthalmos 5.22, 8.25
epiglottic vallecula 5.4
epilepsy 1.28, 2.21, 5.6
Epstein's pearls 4.7
Epstein-Barr virus 2.2, 2.19, 3.13, 5.14
epulis 5.24, 6.8
Erb's palsy 4.3
eruption abnormalities 1.30
eruption cyst 4.17, 8.7
eruption dates 1.7–1.9, 1.29
erythema migrans 3.4, 3.18
extractions/exodontia
   complications 5.5, 5.10, 5.30
   diseases affecting 5.6
   third molars 5.10, 5.16
extrusion 1.5
eye disorders 2.23, 4.2
   fractured orbital floor 5.22, 8.25

facial nerve (CNVII) 3.1, 4.2, 4.3, 5.9, 5.10
facial reconstruction 5.28
facial trauma 5.1–5.2, 5.20–5.22, 8.13–8.14, 8.24–8.25
fear, management of 1.12
felodipine 3.7
fibroepithelial polyp 5.24
fibromyalgia 2.27
fibrosing alveolitis 2.29
fibrous dysplasia 4.24, 8.16–8.17
fluoride 1.21
Fones tooth-brushing technique 1.22
Fordyce's spots 4.7
foreign bodies, inhaled 2.5
fovea palatini 9.1
fractures *see* skull fractures

free flaps 5.28
Frey syndrome 3.26
fungal infections 2.2, 3.5, 4.8
furosemide 7.9

gastric cancer 2.13
gastro-oesophageal reflux disease 2.1, 2.24
Gaucher's disease 4.5
Gengigel 6.24
geographic(al) tongue 3.4, 3.18
giant cell granuloma
   central 8.11–8.12
   peripheral 5.13, 5.24
gingival bleeding 6.8
gingival cyst 4.7
gingival fibromatosis 6.1
gingival hyperplasia 6.8, 6.14
gingivitis 6.7
   ANUG 3.4, 3.5, 6.8, 6.10
gingivostomatitis 1.28, 6.19
Glasgow Coma Scale (GCS) 2.8
glibenclamide 7.8, 7.13
globulomaxillary cyst 4.20
glomerulonephritis 2.10
glossitis 3.4, 3.19
glossopharyngeal nerve (CNIX) 3.1, 4.2
glyceryl trinitrate 7.11, 7.12
gnotobiotic rat study 4.10
gold alloys 9.29
Goltz syndrome 4.5
Gorlin-Goltz syndrome 3.27, 4.19, 8.6
gout 7.27
Gracey curettes 6.2, 6.16
Gram stains 6.20
granular cell myeloblastoma 5.25
Graves' disease 3.26, 4.1, 5.7
Guillain-Barré syndrome 4.1
Gunning splints 5.21

haemochromatosis 2.18
hamular notch 9.1
hand signs 2.26
hang(ing) drop sign 5.22, 8.24
head examination 2.12
headache 3.2, 3.16, 3.17
heart failure 2.5, 2.9, 2.14, 2.18, 2.25, 2.33
Heberden nodes 2.26

Heerfordt syndrome 4.6
hepatic disorders 2.16, 2.18
   and drugs 7.21
hereditary fructose intolerance 4.10
herpes simplex virus 4.4, 5.14
herpes viruses 2.2, 3.13
   see also individual viruses
herpetic gingivostomatitis 1.28, 6.19
histiocytosis 6.4, 6.5
HIV/AIDS 2.2
hoes 6.26
Hopewood House study 4.10
Horner syndrome 2.23, 3.26, 4.3
human papilloma virus 4.4
hydrocolloids 9.30
hypercalcaemia 2.36
hyperparathyroidism 3.24, 8.12
hypertension *see* antihypertensives
hyperthyroidism 2.13, 2.27, 2.36, 3.26, 4.1, 5.7
hyperventilation 2.21, 2.29
hypochlorite 9.17
hypoglossal nerve (CNXII) 3.1, 5.9, 5.10
hypoglycaemia 7.2, 7.10
hypothyroidism 2.11, 2.31, 3.24, 7.2

ibuprofen 5.31, 7.7
ICDAS-II codes 1.4
ileus 2.20
immunoglobulins 6.22
impetigo 1.28, 3.11, 4.4
impression compounds 9.30
incisor angulation/inclination 1.18
index of orthodontic treatment needs (IOTN) 1.20
indirect composites 9.10
infective endocarditis 2.32
inferior alveolar nerve 5.10, 5.16, 5.21
intrusion 1.5, 1.10
isoniazid 7.4
isosorbide mononitrate 7.9

Kaposi's sarcoma 2.2, 3.13, 4.8, 4.26, 5.13
Kennedy classification 9.23
kidney disorders 2.10, 2.16, 2.32, 2.33

INDEX

Laband syndrome 6.1
labial segments 1.18
larynx 5.4
lateral ligament 5.33
lateral pterygoid 5.27
Le Fort classification 5.2
lead poisoning 3.7
Ledermix 9.17
leeway space 1.18
Legionella pneumophila 2.35
leuconychia 2.26
leukaemia 2.19, 6.8
leukoplakia 3.4, 3.8
lichen planus 3.5, 3.23
lignocaine 5.3, 7.4
lipoma 5.25
liver disorders 2.16, 2.18
   and drugs 7.21
long thoracic nerve 4.3
loss of consciousness 2.21, 8.14
lower limb 2.33
Ludwig's angina 5.30
lumps *see* neck lumps; oral lumps/tumours
lung cancer 2.19
lung disorders 2.5, 2.14, 2.29, 2.30, 2.35, 7.16, 7.18
lymphadenopathy 2.19, 3.3, 5.7
lymphoma 5.7

malabsorption 2.13
malar fracture 5.2, 8.13–8.14
malocclusion 1.17, 1.27
mandible 1.24, 8.15
   fracture 5.2, 5.20–5.21
masseter 5.27, 8.14
mastication, muscles 5.27
maxilla 1.24, 5.2
maxillary tuberosity 5.5, 9.1
medial pterygoid 5.27
median rhomboid glossitis 3.4, 3.19
Melkersson-Rosenthal syndrome 3.26
meningism 2.25, 2.32, 3.2
meniscus 5.33
metal alloys 9.29
metastatic cancer 2.15, 2.18
metformin 7.13
methotrexate 6.14, 7.21
metoprolol 7.7
microdontia 1.19
midazolam 7.19
migraine 3.2

mitral stenosis 2.9
Molluscum contagiosum 4.4
moth-eaten bone 8.15
mouth *see entries at* oral
movable joints 9.7
mucocele 4.7, 5.13, 5.23
multiple myeloma 2.10, 4.22, 8.19–8.20
mumps 1.2, 3.6, 5.11, 5.15
muscles of mastication 5.27
myasthenia gravis 4.1
Mycobacterium tuberculosis
   see tuberculosis
mylohyoid ridge 9.1
myocardial infarction 2.7, 2.22, 7.12
myxoma 5.26

nail signs 2.26
nasolabial cyst 4.20
nasopalatine cyst 4.20, 8.18
nasopharynx 5.4
neck examination 2.12
neck lumps 3.3, 5.7
nephritic syndrome 2.33
nerve injury 4.3, 5.10, 5.21
   see also cranial nerves
neurofibromatosis 2.12
neurolemmoma 5.25
nifedipine 6.14
Nikolsky's sign 3.9
Norwalk virus 2.28

occlusion 1.16–1.18, 1.24, 9.14–9.16
   malocclusion 1.17, 1.27
oculomotor nerve (CNIII) 2.23, 4.2, 5.9
odontogenic cysts
   dentigerous 4.16–4.17, 8.7–8.8
   odontogenic keratinocyst 4.18–4.19, 5.16, 8.4, 8.5–8.6
   radicular 4.14–4.15, 8.22
odontogenic tumours 4.12, 4.21, 5.26, 8.4, 8.9–8.10, 8.21, 8.26
odontome 4.21, 5.26, 8.21
oesophagitis 2.22
   reflux 2.1, 2.24
oligodontia 1.19
opiates 7.3
   overdose 2.23, 7.19
oral cancer 5.17, 5.30
   reconstruction 5.28

oral hairy leukoplakia 4.8
oral lumps/tumours 4.7, 5.13, 5.23–5.25, 8.9–8.12, 8.16–8.17, 8.21, 8.26
   see also odontogenic tumours; oral cancer
oral seal 1.16
orbital floor fracture 5.22, 8.24–8.25
orlistat 7.8
oroantral communication 5.5, 5.18–5.19
orofacial granulomatosis 3.20
oropharyngeal anatomy 5.4
oropharyngeal pathology 4.8
Osler nodes 2.26
Osler-Weber-Rendu syndrome 2.12
ossifying fibroma 5.25
osteomyelitis 2.32, 8.15
osteoporosis 2.15
osteosarcoma 4.13
ovarian tumours 2.20
overbite/overjet 1.17
overdose 2.23, 7.19

paediatrics *see entries at* child
Paget's disease 3.28, 4.5, 4.25
pain
   dental 9.12–9.13
   diagnosis 2.15, 2.22, 2.24, 3.2, 3.5
pain relief 5.31, 7.3
   side effects 7.7, 7.8
Papillon-Lefèvre syndrome 4.5, 4.6, 6.4, 6.5, 6.21
paracetamol 7.3, 7.19
parathyroid disease 3.24, 4.5, 8.12
parotid gland 3.3, 5.11, 5.15
Patau syndrome 1.3
Patterson-Brown-Kelly syndrome (Plummer-Vinson) 2.1, 3.27
pellagra 3.4
pellicle 6.7
pemphigoid 3.10
pemphigus 3.9
pepper pot skull 4.22, 8.20
pericarditis/pericardial effusion 2.7
pericoronitis 5.16
PerioChip 6.3, 6.24

INDEX

Periocline 6.3
periodontal abscess 6.13
periodontal examination 6.9, 6.25
periodontal instruments 6.2, 6.16–6.17, 6.26
periodontics 6.1–6.26
   microbiology 6.6–6.7, 6.20
   and systemic disease 6.4–6.5
   treatment 6.3, 6.15–6.16, 6.24
   see also entries at gingiv-
periodontitis 6.4, 6.11–6.12
peripheral neuropathy 4.3, 5.10
peripheral vascular disease 2.33, 5.6
peritonitis 2.20, 2.32
pernicious anaemia 2.6
personality disorders 2.4
pertussis 1.2, 2.5
pharmacology 1.28, 7.1–7.29
   drug interactions 7.20, 7.23
   mechanisms of action 7.9
   side effects 1.31, 3.7, 6.14, 7.4, 7.7–7.8, 7.15, 7.21
   see also antibiotics
pharyngeal pouch 2.1
phenytoin 6.14, 7.4
plaque 6.7
pleomorphic adenoma 5.11, 5.15
pleural effusion 2.14
Plummer–Vinson syndrome 2.1, 3.27
Pneumocystis carinii 2.30, 2.35
pneumonia 2.2, 2.14, 2.29, 2.30, 2.35, 5.30
pneumothorax 2.14
polio 1.2
polyether 9.30
polymyalgia rheumatica 7.27
polypharmacy 7.20, 7.23
polyps 3.5, 5.24
polysulphide 9.30
post-operative complications 5.5, 5.10, 5.30
pre-operative investigations 2.34
pregnancy
   and drugs 5.6, 7.2, 7.24
   epulis 5.24, 6.8
prescriptions 7.17
prilocaine 5.3

primary biliary cirrhosis 4.1
primary survey 5.32
primate space 1.18
probes 6.17
proguanil 3.7
prolactinoma 2.31
prosthodontics see dentures
Pseudomonas aeruginosa 2.35
pulmonary embolism 2.22, 2.25
pulp cap 9.17
pulpitis 9.12, 9.13
pulpotomy 1.25
pyelonephritis 2.32
pyogenic granuloma 5.13, 5.24

radicular cyst 4.14–4.15, 8.22
radiology 8.1–8.26
   equipment 8.3
   frequency 8.1
   views 8.2
radiotherapy 5.16
Ramon syndrome 6.1
Ramsay-Hunt syndrome 3.27
ranula 5.23
reciprocal arms 9.7
reflux oesophagitis 2.1, 2.24
renal colic 2.24, 7.3
renal disorders 2.10, 2.16, 2.32, 2.33
respiratory disorders 2.5, 2.14, 2.29, 2.30, 2.35, 7.16, 7.18
respiratory obstruction 2.5, 5.1
respiratory syncytial virus 2.30
restorative dentistry 9.1–9.30
   anatomy 9.1, 9.21, 9.22
   appearance 9.4
   materials 9.10, 9.17, 9.27–9.30
   preparation 9.8, 9.18
   retention 9.5
   see also dentures
retrobulbar haemorrhage 5.22, 8.25
retromolar pad 9.1
rheumatoid arthritis 7.27
rifampicin 7.21
roll tooth-brushing technique 1.22
root canals 9.21
   treatment 9.18–9.19
root fracture 1.5
root resorption 4.5
root retention 5.30
roseola infantum 3.13

rotavirus 2.28
rubella 1.2
Rutherfurd syndrome 6.1

salbutamol 7.16
salivary glands 3.3, 5.11, 5.15, 8.23
Salmonella 2.28
sarcoidosis 4.6, 5.15
sarin 7.19
scope of practice 9.6
scurvy 2.6, 3.4
sepsis 2.25, 2.32
shingles 3.6, 3.13, 4.4, 5.14
shortness of breath 2.5, 2.29
sialography 8.23
sickles 6.26
silicone 9.30
simvastatin 7.15, 7.21
Sjögren syndrome 3.15, 8.23
skeletal relationships 1.24
skin infections 4.4
skull fractures
   base 5.1
   mandible 5.2, 5.20–5.21
   orbital floor 5.22, 8.24–8.25
   zygoma 5.2, 8.13–8.14
small bowel colic 2.24
small bowel obstruction 2.20
smoking 3.8, 3.19, 5.17, 6.8
solitary bone cyst 4.20
sphenomandibular ligament 5.33
splenomegaly 2.16
splinting of teeth 1.11
squamous cell carcinoma 4.8, 5.17
squamous cell papilloma 5.25
statistics 7.25–7.26
stepdown/stepback techniques 9.18
Stevens–Johnson syndrome 3.27
Stillman tooth-brushing technique 1.6, 1.22
stomach cancer 2.13
stomatitis nicotina 3.8
Streptococcus group A 3.11
Streptococcus pneumoniae 2.30
streptokinase 7.11, 7.12
stroke 2.23
stylomandibular ligament 5.33
subarachnoid haemorrhage 2.21
subluxation 1.10

submandibular gland 3.3
sulphonamides 6.14
supernumerary teeth 1.19, 1.30
supplemental teeth 1.19
surgery 2.34, 5.1–5.33
sutures 5.8, 5.29
syphilis 3.12, 4.23, 5.14
systemic lupus erythematosus (SLE) 2.10, 2.12, 2.19, 3.8

tachycardia 7.28
temporal arteritis 3.2, 3.17
temporalis 5.27
temporomandibular joint dislocation 5.5
tension headache 3.2
tetracycline 1.31
thiazide diuretics 7.1
third molar extraction 5.10, 5.16
thyroglossal cyst 3.3, 5.7
thyroid disease *see* hyperthyroidism; hypothyroidism
tilting casts 9.8
tonsils 5.4
tooth-brushing 1.6, 1.22
tooth mobility index 6.25
tooth reimplantation/ transplantation 1.10
tooth size 1.13, 9.22
tooth surface loss 9.9
toothpaste 9.2

torus 5.13, 5.23
transient ischaemic attack 2.21
trauma
  dental 1.5, 1.10–1.11
  facial 5.1–5.2, 5.20–5.22, 8.13–8.14, 8.24–8.25
  primary survey 5.32
Treponema pallidum 3.12, 4.23, 5.14
tricyclic antidepressants 7.3
trigeminal nerve (CNV) 4.2, 5.9
trigeminal neuralgia 3.2, 3.16
trisomy 21 (Down syndrome) 1.3, 3.27, 6.4, 6.5, 6.18
Tristan da Cunha study 4.10
tuberculosis 1.2, 2.5, 2.13, 2.19, 2.30, 2.35, 5.15
Turku–xylitol study 4.10
Turner syndrome 1.3, 4.5
Turner tooth 1.31

ulcers 5.14
  aphthous 3.5, 3.21–3.22
  duodenal 2.24
  syphilitic 3.12, 4.23, 5.14
uvula 5.4

vagus nerve (CNX) 3.1
varicella zoster virus 3.6, 3.13, 4.4, 5.14
vasovagal faint 2.25
verapamil 7.15

vertebral disc prolapse 2.15
vertebrobasilar ischaemia 2.21
vestibulocochlear nerve (CNVIII) 3.1
vibrating line 5.4
Vipeholm study 4.10
viral infections 1.2, 2.28, 2.30, 2.35, 3.6, 3.13, 4.4, 5.14
  see also specific diseases/ viruses
vitamins
  deficiency 2.6, 3.4
  supplements 7.5
vitiligo pityriasis 2.12
vomiting 2.28
Von Recklinghausen syndrome 3.27

warfarin 7.15
Wegener granulomatosis 2.27
weight loss 2.13
white spongy naevus 3.8
WHO probes 6.17
whooping cough 1.2, 2.5
Williams probes 6.17
wisdom tooth extraction 5.10, 5.16
working lengths 9.22

X-rays *see* radiology
xerostomia 3.15

zinc oxide paste 9.30
zygoma fracture 5.2, 8.13–8.14